Behind Closed Doors

Morality and Society Series

EDITED BY ALAN WOLFE

Recent Titles:

For a complete list of series titles, please see the end of the book.

Behind Closed Doors

IRBs and the Making of Ethical Research

LAURA STARK

The University of Chicago Press
Chicago and London

Laura Stark is assistant professor of science in society and of sociology at Wesleyan University.

The University of Chicago Press, Chicago 60637
The University of Chicago Press, Ltd., London
© 2012 by The University of Chicago
All rights reserved. Published 2012.
Printed in the United States of America

21 20 19 18 17 16 15 14 13 12   1 2 3 4 5

ISBN-13: 978-0-226-77086-4 (cloth)
ISBN-13: 978-0-226-77087-1 (paper)
ISBN-10: 0-226-77086-9 (cloth)
ISBN-10: 0-226-77087-7 (paper)

Library of Congress Cataloging-in-Publication Data

Stark, Laura Jeanine Morris, 1975–
    Behind closed doors : IRBs and the making of ethical research / Laura Stark.
        p. cm. — (Morality and society series)
    Includes bibliographical references and index.
    ISBN-13: 978-0-226-77086-4 (cloth: alk. paper)
    ISBN-10: 0-226-77086-9 (cloth: alk. paper)
    ISBN-13: 978-0-226-77087-1 (pbk.: alk. paper)
    ISBN-10: 0-226-77087-7 (pbk.: alk. paper)   1. Institutional review
boards (Medicine)—United States—History. 2. Human experimentation in
medicine—Government policy—United States. 3. Medical ethics—United
States—History—20th century. 4. Research—Moral and ethical aspects—
United States. 5. Research—Government policy—United States.   I. Title.
II. Series: Morality and society.
    R852.5S837 2012
    174.2'8—dc22

                                                        2011013642

♾ This paper meets the requirements of ANSI/NISO Z39.48-1992
(Permanence of Paper).

For Gary and Vi Morris

CONTENTS

Behind Closed Doors

Governing with Experts

In 1961 the town of Bethesda, Maryland, was—as it is today—a quiet, afflu-ent suburb of Washington, D.C. Thus, it may have seemed improbable to residents that two federal prisoners awoke near the golf course on January 6 of that year and left town in time to catch a midmorning flight out of the Washington airport.[1]

The prisoners had been neighbors of a sort. That winter, the two men lived in Bethesda just off Wisconsin Avenue at the National Institutes of Health (NIH) research hospital, called the Clinical Center. Throughout the 1960s, the federal government moved men from penitentiaries across the country to the Clinical Center for several weeks or months at a time, most often in groups of twenty-five. They stayed in wards set aside for the study of infectious diseases and pulled off only a few "unauthorized leaves," the phrase that NIH leaders used to refer to events that were more colloqui-ally known as escapes.[2] Throughout the 1960s, NIH researchers infected them either with malaria or with viral diseases: pneumonia, flu, or an illness caused by simian virus-40. Research on prisoners was common in the United States at the time, and American scientists worked hard to craft domestic and international ethics standards—the 1964 Declaration of Helsinki, for example—that allowed them to continue prisoner research.[3] Although com-monly done and formally allowed, prisoner research was still contentious. Sensing this, NIH leaders made sure the prisoner program remained "little known to the general public," as the surgeon general phrased it in 1964. Even within the Clinical Center, it struck some NIH doctors, lawyers, and administrators as somehow wrong to infect and study prisoners. But despite their misgivings, they went along with research practices that worried them.

Lawyers who were personally uneasy nonetheless endorsed the research in their professional role as legal counsel to the U.S. government. Likewise, doctors who felt troubled made peace, eventually, with their colleagues' practices.

At NIH in the postwar decades, research that might have prompted controversy quietly proceeded because the leaders of the Clinical Center had collectively agreed on a method for recognizing a good, fair decision about whether research was acceptable. If a study was endorsed by a particular group of scientists, called the Clinical Research Committee, the study became acceptable. The committee, in effect, defined whether studies were proper. This was procedure, and—in the case of the prisoners' study and in thousands of studies since—research went ahead because procedure had been followed. In this case, like many others, ethics rules served to enable research as much as to restrict it.[4]

This book explores how researchers designed U.S. government rules for the treatment of human subjects after World War II, and it examines the present-day consequences of their choice to adopt review procedures rather than ethics principles. NIH leaders built and defended rules that they felt suited their particular circumstances. In so doing they invented a new federal standard for how courts, colleagues, and research participants would learn to recognize ethical research. In the decades since the Clinical Center opened in 1953, there have been profound changes in the scope, funding, and ethics of research on human subjects. But what has endured is a way of making research ethical, a method of "governing with experts." In the name of federal law, groups of individuals thought to have unique qualifications approve (or reject) researchers' choices about who should participate and how participants should be studied. In the process, they also shape research because they are empowered by law to require changes to studies before they approve them. More often than not, expert groups do exercise their legal authority to request modifications. Whether that involves editing the questions researchers ask in a survey or trimming the number of patients that doctors enroll in a clinical trial, review boards help to create today's biomedical and social science research.[5]

NIH doctors, lawyers, and administrators adopted this method of governing with experts to manage research inside the NIH Clinical Center in the years when words like *Sputnik*, *double helix*, and *McCarthyism* entered common parlance. They did not anticipate at the time that their particular local arrangement would endure. Yet it became the model for human-subjects review boards, and its legacy is with us today wherever scientists and scholars plan to study human beings.

Rule Experts and Knowledge Experts

Part of the role of government agencies is to empower people to make decisions on behalf of the people being governed. Whereas some laws are in place to keep order among citizens, another set of rules—administrative law—guides the daily work of government employees. The point of the rules is to enable civil servants to make rote, seemingly impersonal decisions in our stead. In theory, the rules are so precise that they would allow all qualified people to reach the same conclusion.[6] Administrative laws are designed to make human decisions appear to be objective and beyond the judgment of a given individual.

This imperative of objectivity surrounds us. Think of food inspectors, drug regulators, and housing authorities. Imagine the mindless rule-follower conjured by the cliché that decisions are made by "some bureaucrat in Washington."[7] The rules that civil servants apply are often quantified: calorie counts, chemical ratios, and rating scores, for example. The paradox is that qualities of human experience that would not otherwise be thought of numerically—the seeming intangibles and passions of learning, loving, and living in general—are often quantified when inserted into regulatory apparatuses *so that* rules can be applied.[8] Civil servants become agile in using a narrow set of regulations, and gradually, in the course of doing their jobs, they become *rule experts.*

Most citizens are limited not only by time but also by the knowledge needed to make informed collective decisions. None of us know all of the things needed to participate meaningfully in each decision that affects us, and, frankly, neither do civil servants. For this work, governments turn to *knowledge experts.*[9]

Government agencies outsource decision making to people who are already trained in specialist areas. Groups of experts in science, law, medicine, and other fields of formal knowledge have been tapped to do the everyday work of applying administrative laws to concrete cases. During the 1960s, the U.S. Congress passed an unprecedented number of federal statutes that dramatically expanded the scope of federal programs, and these programs were overwhelmingly aimed at regulating the natural environment and human health. As a result, specialists in these fields have been incorporated in growing numbers into the process of writing and applying regulations.[10] Academics, for example, decide which medicines are safe to study and prescribe, how much doctors get paid through Medicaid, and which artists, scholars, scientists, and businesses are worth supporting with public money.[11]

These people are what anthropologist Donald Brenneis calls "nonce bureaucrats." They are bureaucrats only temporarily and for a specific decision-making purpose.[12] Their full-time jobs are elsewhere, often doing whatever it is that makes them knowledge experts in the first place, such as practicing law, researching chemical compounds, or studying scripture. They are called on to make decisions that defy strict, quantifiable rules—decisions that call instead for judgment.

Administrative laws empower knowledge experts to make seemingly idiosyncratic decisions. For rule experts, use of discretion would be an abuse of power; but for knowledge experts it is their mandate. Legal scholar Duncan Kennedy argues that discretion has been built into rational—that is to say, rule-bound—decision-making practices in modern democratic governments. In many cases, making value judgments is not antithetical to following the official rules but is precisely what it means to follow the letter of the law. The value of nonce bureaucrats to governments is their apparent ability to use discretion soundly, not to avoid discretion altogether.[13]

Declarative Bodies

But knowledge experts create a problem of their own. If democratic decisions are supposed to be beyond the caprice of an individual, how can we be sure that an expert uses her discretion to arrive at an objective (read *fair and democratic*) decision?[14] The answer is that legitimate discretionary decisions have to be made by a group: a body of multiple experts.[15] Citizens, of course, have to abide by these choices, which are often made in seclusion in settings that, if not formally restricted to the public, are at least cumbersome to access. And while we may protest, resist, or appeal their group decisions, doing so would work against the grain of the status quo, which these bodies have the authority to set.

That is to say, their words matter. Administrative law gives certain people the authority, in specific contexts, to change our shared reality. The classic example of how some people's words have special power is that of a justice of the peace saying "I now pronounce you legally married." He is not describing a married couple; rather, he is creating one. For these words to stick—that is, for other people to treat the pair as a married couple, both legally and socially—the setting has to be appropriate (e.g., spoken when all three are present), and everyone else has to agree that the authority figure has the power he claims (i.e., that he can marry people). Then, as if by magic, people's financial, legal, and social worlds can change.

It is the same with the entities I call *declarative bodies*.[16] I use this term to demarcate groups of knowledge experts who are empowered by law to make decisions for citizens. The say-so of these declarative bodies has tangible, material consequences. For example, the Federal Reserve Board decided which institutions American taxpayers would keep afloat in the 2008 financial crisis, and the Medicare Payment Advisory Commission tells doctors how much they will get paid for seeing low-income patients. The decisions of these expert groups are just words, and yet those words have the power to change the world in which we live.

One type of declarative body decides whether research on people can proceed. These groups are called institutional review boards (IRBs), and their archetype was the Clinical Research Committee developed at NIH. Today, an IRB is supposed to sign off on any study that uses "human subjects" before it can take place, whether the researcher plans to observe participants in a community meeting or to test a new drug on children. IRBs decide who may and may not be studied and what may and may not be done to people in various circumstances. IRBs are declarative bodies because they are empowered to turn a hypothetical situation (this study *may be* acceptable) into shared reality (this study *is* acceptable). It is a testament to the power of their words that IRBs rarely disapprove studies but regularly change them. In so doing they change what is knowable.

IRBs in Practice

Almost all hospitals, universities, and other organizations that support research on people have IRBs, including private companies and government agencies. Today, the federal government counts nearly four thousand boards in the United States alone, and thousands more abroad. Their ubiquity is no coincidence: federal law requires that nearly all research on people be vetted by a review board before it begins.[17] Traditionally, IRBs have been housed within these institutions (hence the name *institutional* review board). Recently, though, private IRBs have cropped up, unattached to any "institution" per se. They are freestanding corporations that review studies for a fee. After all, to make an IRB you just need five experts, a record-keeping system, and the blessing of the federal Office for Human Research Protections, and this has left room for creative variation.

What we know about IRBs comes, primarily, from survey data and from firsthand accounts written by researchers whose proposals have undergone review.[18] These sources have helped to create the general impression that

IRBs work slowly, demand study changes often, and are largely administrative.[19] Fair enough.

In addition to being a troublesome part of researchers' daily grind, however, IRBs are also an example of a type of declarative body that fits into a wider system of governing with experts. Like other declarative bodies, IRBs have wide latitude in making decisions, so long as they make choices together. This social arrangement sets up a number of puzzles. For example, how do experts resolve disagreements, if each member has a claim to special knowledge? What sustains the impression that these people, together, are one uniquely empowered social actor? What, in sum, do knowledge experts take into account in their meetings behind closed doors?

I take up these questions in part 1 of this book, using IRBs as my example of a declarative body. Chapters 1, 2, and 3 are based on IRB meetings that I watched, audio-recorded, and analyzed at three sites for a stretch of time that ranged from several months (in the case of one medical board) to a full year (in the cases of two boards at different research-intensive state universities). I also interviewed the members of these boards and the chairs of different IRBs across the country, though I did not contact researchers or research participants, because of confidentiality concerns. (For more details, please see the appendix.) Appropriately enough, I had to get approval from IRBs at Princeton University and NIH for the research I did for this book. As I have come to know more about IRBs, they have become an avocation for me, as well.[20]

What I offer is a perspective from inside IRB meetings from the vantage point of a curious observer with no stake in the decision outcomes. What I learned was that the *techniques* IRB members used to reach decisions were strikingly similar at these different locations. To be clear, the IRBs I studied reached very different conclusions about similar studies. No surprise: they were working in different settings, were composed of quite different individuals, and made ample use of their discretionary prerogative.

But their methods for reaching decisions were patterned: board members tended to read researchers' application documents like tea leaves for signs of good character; to use *warrants* for expertise to justify their recommendations; to invoke previous decisions they had made as *local precedents* to guide future decisions; and, ingeniously, to use meeting minutes to manage relationships among board members and between board members and researchers under review.

Without planning or communicating, the various IRBs reached decisions using similar methods, and this, I argue, is a product of their common configuration. Starting in 1966, the U.S. surgeon general required all institutions that hosted research on people to get prior approval from a human-subjects review committee. This included universities, hospitals, and other organizations; and it covered both biomedical and social scientists. If the research was attached to public money, then this new policy was attached to the research. The model acquired teeth in 1974 when the Congress enacted regulation that required prior review (specifically, the National Research Act). The review model that was outlined in the 1966 policy and strengthened in the 1974 regulations came directly out of NIH.[21]

To understand how boards work today requires knowing how the research review model developed at NIH. How, for example, did expert deliberation come to be regarded as a sensible way to ensure upstanding research? Why did thousands of IRBs pop up at sites across the country, when the function could have been handled by a single federal IRB, as advocates urged, or by several regional boards, as in the UK?[22]

The story of how IRBs work is a story about their past, as well as their present. Typically, the origins of IRBs are explained through a series of scandals. The standard narrative often starts with the Nazi medical experiments during World War II. These atrocities prompted the 1947 Nuremberg Code, which set down on paper the ten moral imperatives that its American authors claimed all ethical researchers, like themselves, already knew. Twenty-five years later, the revelation of the long-running Tuskegee Syphilis Study on black men in rural Alabama triggered the National Research Act, which empowered the federal government to regulate research on people. The act also mandated a statement of principles on research ethics, which is known today as the Belmont Report. Casting further back, various accounts recall how doctors avoided misdeeds by observing the Hippocratic Oath; or explain how the 1930 vaccine tragedy in Lübeck, Germany, prompted research regulations even before the Nazis came to power; or recount how in 1966 Dr. Henry K. Beecher bravely exposed research abuses within his own profession.[23] Starting in 2010, future histories will add the intentional-infection experiments on Guatemalans, who were given syphilis in the 1940s by American researchers.[24]

In the history of ethics, accounts of research scandals serve many purposes. They reveal the terms of political debate and the stakeholders relevant at a given time and place. Scandals serve as object lessons—shared memories with a moral, which are meant to teach people a common ethical sense in the present day. Careful histories of scandals also show how difficult it is to cast pure heroes and villains. Such accounts are important in that they can prompt political change and indicate the contours of a collective conscience.

One aim of this book, however, is to explain the content of political and intellectual changes. As a result, what I call critical-event narratives are less of a driving force in the chapters that follow than they are in other studies of research ethics. Instead, I explore how it came to be that groups of experts seemed well suited to make important choices about people's rights. In chapters 4, 5, and 6, I explain how the moral authority to decide how to treat research participants was relocated from professions to the state and reinvested in procedures rather than ethics principles. I show how the practice of committee review within the NIH Clinical Center was created in the early 1950s to manage the unvarnished reality that NIH was hospitalizing healthy American civilians, in addition to sick patients, for medical research. The problems NIH leaders fretted over derived as much from a new kind of doctor, the "physician-researcher," as from a new kind of patient, the "healthy patient." In an effort to outflank federal lawyers and manage practical problems, researchers inside the Clinical Center developed a committee review system.[25] The practice of expert review (or at least its rhetoric) was further entrenched in the late 1950s and early 1960s by researchers at the core of American biomedicine.

The model of group review was invented, justified, and expanded less by "outsiders" like bioethicists and activists than by the researchers themselves. The language of bioethics that has been read back into the history of IRBs belies their past as a technique for promoting research and preventing lawsuits. At NIH expert-review boards were crafted as an alternative to professional codes of ethics, which adhered to practitioners rather than to places of research. In contrast to the history often recounted in the bioethics literature, I give an on-the-ground story that shows how changes in the patronage of science affected research practices and moral sensibilities.

Because they bear the vestiges of this origin, IRBs today can enable surprising research practices. At the same time, they can restrict research in uneven ways. There is no dispute that the current research review system is flawed. On this everyone agrees: board members, administrators, and researchers. But the fact that IRBs provoke such heated debate is all the more reason to understand how these declarative bodies came into being and how they actually do their work. And so, on a dreary May afternoon, I stepped out of an elevator at Adams University Medical School, walked down a windowless corridor, and opened the conference room door where the IRB meeting was about to begin.

PART I

IRBs in Action

There are things IRB members are supposed to do: assess risks and safeguard participants' rights. Board members say that they do these things because they are moral imperatives and also because they are the law.

Then there are things IRB members do by virtue of the social arrangement created through these laws. It is hard for a group of people to assess the risks of research and safeguard the rights of participants while seated at a conference table, particularly when two crucial people are absent from the meeting rooms: namely, the researcher and the research participant. Researchers are absent from most IRB meetings by custom. Research participants are missing by definition: people cannot be recruited for research until after the IRB has approved recruiting them. Without the researcher and the subject, how do these decisions get made?

The chapters in part 1 take up this question and answer it in different but complementary ways. The aim of this introduction is to give a sense of what IRB meetings look like from the inside before showing how IRB members make decisions. My view is not the same one you will get from reading ethics training manuals. This is not to say that the IRB members at Adams, Greenly, and Sander State University were deviant or that their meetings went off script.[1] The point, rather, is that IRB members have shared understandings about how to do their work, which they do not need to articulate. Their tacit understandings are in the background of the discussions that are on display in the subsequent chapters.

The Balancing Act

IRBs deliberate over a particular subset of studies during what is called full-board review. These were the types of reviews I observed in the meetings I attended.[2] Generally speaking, studies that are regarded as especially sensitive—potentially dangerous or possibly coercive ones, for example—are the studies that all the board members evaluate together, regardless of the research method. In addition to studies that receive full-board review, IRB administrators can place submissions in two other categories: "exempt" and "expedited." The administrator or a few members can evaluate these studies independently.[3]

According to federal regulation, the people who carry out full-board review have to fit a general mold. In terms of membership, IRBs must include at least five people. Some may have as many as twenty. The boards I observed averaged ten. The bulk of the members are supposed to represent "expertise" in the areas in which investigators propose to conduct their research, although no board member who is actually involved in the study under review may vote on it. There must be at least one board member who is *not* affiliated with the institution, and one member must have "nonscientific" concerns. Operationally, these requirements are often taken to mean that these members should not hold an advanced degree. In some cases, however, these members (sometimes referred to as "community members" or "community representatives") do have formal research training, as was the case for doctors in private practice and theologians who served on the boards I observed.[4] The National Bioethics Advisory Commission has recommended that one-quarter of IRB members should be community representatives and one-quarter should not be affiliated with the institution, but most IRBs fall short of this ideal.[5] The federal government strongly urges that boards include at least one man and one woman, and it more gently encourages that members of racial minority groups be included on the boards, though the regulations do not, strictly speaking, set quotas for the race and gender composition of boards.[6] As of 2002, one-quarter of IRBs had memberships that were exclusively white, and seven out of ten IRBs had male majorities.[7] Within these flexible guidelines, local IRBs have the latitude to develop different standards and practices.

All members of the IRBs I observed had been appointed by a university administrator (e.g., the vice president for research); many saw themselves as fulfilling a service requirement; and a few had negotiated stipends or, for faculty members, course release.[8] Most IRB members with whom I spoke reported that they served because they personally enjoyed it or because they wanted to serve as a "proresearch" presence on what is commonly considered a restrictive committee at universities. Perhaps institutions make the most of the resonance of "ethics work" with other kinds of activities that are thought to be altruistic but become morally suspect if money changes hands: for example, donating blood, organs, or ova. By referring to board members' work as a gift—in their case, a gift of time—their choices can be made to seem more ethical and good. In any event, the board members whom I observed overwhelmingly described their group as very "compatible" and "collegial," despite differences in training and personal background. This is no coincidence: members of declarative bodies tend to be selected not only for what they know and whom they represent, but also for a capacity that anthropologist Donald Brenneis calls "amiable mutual deference," which smooths the deliberative process.[9] The group members I observed worked to be accommodating of each other, in part because of this selection bias and also because board members get authority from federal regulations insofar as they act in unison as "the IRB."

There are three moral principles—respect for persons, beneficence, and justice—that, in theory, guide IRB members' interpretation of the nuts and bolts of regulations. When the Congress passed the National Research Act in 1974, it required that a national commission be created to review and ideally improve the laws for human-subjects protections that had just been enacted. That body, formally called the National Commission for the Protection of Human Subjects of Biomedical and Behavioral Research, worked hard on many thorny issues (e.g., prison research) for many long years. One of their final acts, required by the 1974 law, was to articulate guiding principles for research on human subjects. In 1979 they published the Belmont Report (named for the conference center where the group met) to outline the overarching spirit in which the regulations should be interpreted. The commissioners decided that the three principles would come into play in three corollary practices: making sure that the people being studied were not chosen in discriminatory ways; ensuring that participants had adequate information when they agreed to be studied; and ensuring that the risks to participants (whether physical, social, or legal) were appropriate in light of the potential benefits of the study, either for the participants or for others. The shorthand for this final task, according to the Belmont Report, was to weigh risks and benefits. For IRB members, weighing risks and benefits of a study is a daunting task, in part because the commissioners themselves regarded it as an aspiration that could never fully be achieved.[10]

Why three principles, you might ask, and not four or four hundred? Sociologist John Evans has explained that this was a somewhat arbitrary choice but that it is a brand of arbitrariness that works well for modern liberal governments, in which the most seemingly impersonal decisions are taken to be the most legitimate.[11] One way to make decisions seem impersonal is to use rational—that is to say, highly rule-bound—decision-making techniques. Since the 1930s, rational decision making has taken the form of "balancing"—or cost-benefit analysis in one incarnation.[12] It was not inevitable that cost-benefit analysis would become the main tool of rational regulatory decision making, but it has nonetheless become "the dominant logic of government."[13] The aim is to encourage people acting on behalf of the government, whether they are rule experts or knowledge experts, to make decisions that either are based on numbers or seem to be.

As a result, the language of weighing risks against benefits is pervasive among IRB members, but board member rarely do—or even are able to—use quantitative balancing in any practical sense. In the 1970s, even the members of the National Commission recognized the "metaphorical character of these terms." Given that IRB members have (and use) a good deal of discretion when they evaluate researchers' studies, it may be reassuring to know that the commissioners themselves felt that "only on rare occasions" would "quantitative techniques be available for the scrutiny of research protocols." That said, the commissioners nonetheless felt that "the idea of systematic, nonarbitrary analysis of risks and benefits should be emulated insofar as possible." The point of emulating a quantitative technique in what they acknowledged was an inherently qualitative assessment was to make the review "more rigorous and precise, while making communication between review board members and investigators less subject to misinterpretation, misinformation and conflicting judgments." The commission's advice to IRB members—that they metaphorically weigh risks and benefits—may have had an effect precisely opposite to the one they intended.[14]

The metaphor of weighing risks and benefits has come to serve many purposes in IRB meetings. At a Greenly IRB meeting, for example, the rhetoric of risk-benefit analysis oriented board members' thinking in the broadest sense and also added humor, irony, and reflexivity to reviews. In one case, a researcher recently hired by the university submitted a protocol for a study funded through the American Heart Association that involved enrolling older men at risk of a heart attack. Board members felt the researcher's protocol was too short ("a précis"), his information for participants too technical ("is it too much for a consent to be understandable?"), and his general demeanor "cavalier" ("He's from [another research university]. Maybe they're less demanding there.")[15] More broadly, this lax kind of researcher was, in the board chair's estimation, an example of how the university was "getting new faculty, who are also very oriented to this type of protocol." One board member, Nathan, a reluctant bioethicist who preferred to avoid the tinge of righteousness by describing himself as just a member of the philosophy department, was concerned that these new researchers were not restrictive enough in their exclusion requirements for heart patients. A change to the research design would be entirely fair for board members to request, they decided, trying to shoehorn their good sense into the balancing metaphor. Here is an excerpt of the meeting that shows how IRB members use the rhetoric of weighing when deciding issues that do not register on scales. This excerpt also introduces some of the conventions that ethnographers use to designate in texts how people's conversations sound in real time. (For a list of transcription conventions and their meanings, please see the appendix.)

CHAIR (UNIVERSITY RESEARCH ADMINISTRATION): Nathan raises an interesting point because one of the things we are charged with doing is to determine whether the risk [is worth the—
EDWARD (FACULTY, ARCHITECTURE): Risk is worth the benefit.]
CHAIR: Whether the uh =
DR. MORRIS (OUTSIDE PHYSICIAN): Benefit is worth the risk.
NATHAN (FACULTY, PHILOSOPHY-BIOETHICS): *h* Something like that.[16]

The language of weighing risks and benefits is more rhetorically useful, perhaps, than actual attempts to compare incommensurable things. Above all, it serves the purpose of demonstrating that a decision maker knows the rules of the game. Members of declarative bodies invoke regulatory language to show that they are aware of what they are doing, especially when they use their discretion to interpret the rules creatively.

Seeing Like a Subject

The people who do the day-to-day work of governing—who decide where to build a dam, a dump, or a sidewalk, for example—have a tendency, within some systems of government, to see only physical resources and the interests of power holders when they are preparing to make a decision. They tend not to see—not to imagine—the tangible consequences of their decisions for individual people on the ground who may be affected. Historian James Scott has called this phenomenon "seeing like a state."[17] Within the legal systems of modern liberal democracies, the people who do the day-to-day work of governing are encouraged also to "see like a subject." In other words, rule experts and knowledge experts enact regulations that require them to imagine the perspectives of people whom the law is controlling or safeguarding. From the vantage point of a research institution, seeing like a subject is a way to reduce the chances that subjects will have reason to sue, which they are empowered to do, based on laws such as human-subjects regulations.

One example of how regulations encourage IRB members to see like a subject is in locating the crucial threshold between studies that present "no more than minimal risk" to participants and more risky studies. The distinction hinges on whether the study presents greater social, legal, or physical risks than a participant would experience in her everyday life. The question for board members, then, is what the participant's everyday life is like, and whether the research involves experiences and procedures that are much different. If so, then the burden is on the researcher to show greater benefit.

What are the experiences of would-be research participants in their everyday lives, and how can you know? Previous studies on courts and on state administration would suggest that IRB members might think of research participants in the aggregate and of individual participants as microcosms of the broader population to which they belong.[18] This was not the case among board members, though. To make decisions in IRB meetings, board members imagined the people who featured in their own lives as stand-ins for research participants. During an IRB meeting at Greenly, for example, an anthropologist on the board argued that children answering one researcher's proposed questionnaire would experience it as "invasive" because of the racial experiences of one of his own students. Earlier in the day, the student had told the anthropologist about how "when [the student] was two years old he was given a real hard time because he was sort of dark skinned but not quite clear. And he was being told, `Are you black or white?' That is a good bit of concern. [Participants] should know that this is what kind of questions [they're] going to get."[19] At another meeting, a sports coach on the board insisted that a researcher change the information that he was planning to give participants in a bone-density study. At issue was how best to express the risk of radiation exposure so that participants could consent with full information. That board member disliked the researcher's plan to express the radiation dosage relative to the amount from getting an X-ray: "When you say it's going to be / that it's the same as a normal X-ray—I mean, I can see my father going, `How much radiation is that?' "[20]

The people whom board members called to mind when they imagined a research subject—a relative or a student, for example—reinforced the race, class, and gender biases of the board membership. This often took place, paradoxically, during the review of studies that aimed to question conventional wisdom about health, social groups, and human experience.

Ambiguities over the boundaries of the groups that IRB members saw themselves as protecting and representing—that is, the slipperiness of terms like *community* and *population* in IRB meetings—created situations in which all IRB members could usefully explain how their own life experiences might help the board more fully imagine the perspective of potential research subjects. At one meeting, for example, confusion over study recruitment snowballed because, a board member pointed out, it was unclear whether the phrase, "the control group will be recruited from the community" meant that the investigator would be "recruiting people here on the campus," whether she would be "really looking at heart patients, the community of heart patients in this case," or whether she would recruit from "the general community."[21] This same ambiguity over the meaning of *community* is inherent in the role of "community members" on the board. All IRB members could interject their opinions and warrants for their views through their claims to knowledge about participants by thinking of their friends, family members, students, neighbors, colleagues, and acquaintances. In this way, the membership of the IRB informs who is called to mind when board members imagine a research participant. (For more on the warrant of personal experience, see chapter 1.)

It is fair to say that neither researchers nor IRB members can know how each potential research participant will feel about the risks of a study or the adequacy of information about it. Given that people change their minds and often feel ambivalent, it is also fair to expect that participants' own feelings about serving in a study will not be stable. As a result, the aim of human-subjects regulations (and in particular, the notion of informed consent) is to get potential research participants also to recognize *themselves* as "human subjects," a legal category invented in the 1960s that now tends to be used to refer to anyone who participates in research. In sum, the review system aims to make sure that when researchers are studying people, each participant has come to see himself like a subject and that IRB members think of participants not in terms of populations, but as analogues of specific, tangible people whom they know in their daily lives.[22]

Housekeeping Work

Quotidian as it is, research review often boils down to paperwork. To be sure, administrators do the thankless work of tracking and filing applications, forms, and e-mails between researchers and reviewers. But IRB members also deal with paperwork in a very different but nonetheless important way.

IRB members use the documents that researchers send to the board to judge the character of the researchers. For board members, the style and tidiness of researchers' documents offer a snapshot of the person behind the application.[23] Since researchers are invited to IRB meetings to talk about their studies at only 10 percent of American boards, the self-portrait that a researcher presents in her paperwork is often the only glimpse that board members get.

At Sander State, the board members liked to use the term *housekeeping* to refer to a particular kind of work they did during meetings—as in "There are a couple of housekeeping issues. The informed consent needs to identify this as a [Sander State University] study right up top" or (from a different member at the same meeting) "I have just a housekeeping issue here. The students are listed as co-investigators when actually they should be listed as key personnel."[24] IRB members used the term *housekeeping* to refer to a type of paperwork that was a chore. No one relished making such changes, but they had to be made, like it or not: fixing typographical errors, correcting formatting glitches, and making other changes to produce clean documents.

When they did housekeeping work, however, board members and administrators were doing something essential to the review process. They were evaluating the researcher. It was through their reading and visual inspection of the documents, such as protocols, consent forms, and recruitment fliers, that board members developed their sense of whether they trusted the researcher. Since IRB members cannot oversee all studies as they are carried out, the group must be willing to trust that investigators are fastidious. When board members had reservations about a researcher, they gave the IRB a stronger presence in the research, for example by requiring that the researcher report to the board more frequently than is required by regulation or by selecting the study for an IRB audit.

Thus ink and paper served as character witnesses. At Greenly IRB, for example, one board member, Dr. Morris, who was a head administrator at a local hospital, chided a researcher who misspelled "principal" in the subject heading of his protocol. In an interview after the meeting, I asked Dr. Morris to tell me how he goes about reviewing protocols when they come across his desk. Among other things, he volunteered that he looks for "misspellings" and other "editorial things" which "bother" him because such shortcomings demonstrate "a lack of attention to detail." Then he told me about the peanut butter phenomenon:

> It's that old phrase, you never get a second chance to make a first impression. . . . I think that it colors the impression of the reviewer immediately. . . . One of my old professors, a long, long time ago, who was an internationally

known reviewer, called it the peanut butter phenomenon. He said that invariably when he got things to review, he would always find that somebody had spilled—this was twenty or thirty years ago—somebody had spilled some food on it and then left it. . . . And he said, "This person has insulted me by not retyping the page even though they spilled their peanut butter and jelly sandwich." And so that was like an automatic "gone." You know, in the wastebasket. And I always remember him describing that, and I guess it's the extension of the peanut butter phenomenon. This is a person who's not careful enough to make sure that the word is spelled right.[25]

Why, specifically, is sloppiness relevant for research review? For Dr. Morris, "If [a researcher's] attention to detail is not sufficient to know that the major heading, the words aren't spelled right, I'm worried about [other things as well like], do I have to read this thing carefully enough to make sure that all the doses, for example, are correct, that they've written the protocol correctly. [I wonder] where else is it sloppy? You know, four micrograms of nitroglycerin instead of point-four or four hundred micrograms of nitroglycerin. I mean, how careful do I have to be?"[26] Similarly, a historian on the Sander State IRB described herself as "a stickler for detail" in protocol reviews. In addition to issues of confidentiality, she said, she was particularly attuned to "any inconsistency in the protocols, any of the specifics." She explained: "If it is an excessively sloppy proposal, I'm going to be more questioning about it. Even if the researcher thinks [the study] is potentially valuable, I do think they should be made to take care, take the time, get it right. . . . I would be prejudiced against it if it is full of typos, inconsistencies, factual errors that would make me doubt. I'd be questioning about the ability of the researcher."[27] Board members parlayed the researcher's apparent attention to detail in documents into judgments of professional competence.

This was also apparent in meetings of the Adams Medical IRB. The university was in the process of replacing its old paper-based submission system with a new computerized system that allowed investigators to submit their IRB documents online. When errors appeared in investigators' documents—a recurring topic of conversation at the meetings—the board members did not simply note that the investigator needed to resubmit the materials. Instead, they tried to figure out who or what was to blame for the error: the investigator or the software. For example, after an IRB member, Dr. G, presented to the board what she regarded as a generally "weak" proposal, her comments begged the question of responsibility:

DR. G: [Overall, the proposal] needs to be much more clearly stated.

DR. K: Is this just a [software] error where they—

DR. G: I don't know. Don't know. It's a very, very brief protocol, so—I know [the investigator] quite well. She was on call on this Saturday, and I was hoping /

IRB CHAIR: I think it's not a [software] thing. Yeah, it's not a [software] thing.

DR. G: It's a submission thing.

IRB CHAIR: Yeah.[28]

Board members were interested to know whether the software was causing problems so that the flaws in the system could be repaired (although there was a full-time staff member at the university whose job was to do just this). But determining responsibility for administrative errors also suggested to members of the Adams Medical IRB whether the researcher was properly supervising a study—giving subordinates too much responsibility or being careless when signing off on documents written in his name. Seemingly mundane aspects of the IRB review process are unusually important precisely because board members consider them appropriate grounds for judging the quality and integrity of investigators, whereas ascribed characteristics like race and gender cannot be used to judge researchers (though these factors are taken into account in selecting members of the IRB).[29]

Housekeeping work also helps to explain a curious feature of IRB meetings: when a researcher whose study is under review is also sitting at the table (or is on the other end of a conference call), then the review process is faster, not slower. Studies have found that the number of days between submitting a protocol and getting final approval is shorter when the investigator is present—even if the meetings themselves are not shorter by the standards of a stopwatch. In addition, when researchers attend meetings, there are fewer documents exchanged between researchers and board members: fewer letters, e-mails, and drafts of forms and protocols.[30] When researchers are not present, IRB members not only invest more time in housekeeping work (and, ironically, demand more documents); they also use researchers' paper trails to predict whether the researchers will follow the protocol laid out and actually prevent risks, protect rights, and deflect lawsuits.

Conclusion

IRB members were very good with worst-case scenarios. Supposedly, Americans have an easier time imagining good outcomes than bad ones, down to the finest detail. Ideal scenarios are somehow reinvented in the mind's eye as the most plausible outcomes. But this tends not to be the case for IRB members.[31]

The difference may rest with the fact that board members were not thinking about their personal futures during meetings. They were not discussing eventualities that were mostly within their control. Rather, board members were handed specific details about a future scenario that a researcher would be guiding and that would affect yet-unknown research participants. Strictly speaking, the task of IRB members during full-board review is to evaluate two things: whether researchers plan to observe participants' rights (typically through "informed consent") and whether researchers plan to keep any risks to participants in proportion to the expected benefits of the study. And yet board members have to be inventive in making decisions about people who are not present: researchers and participants. As a result, they made decisions through metaphorical "balancing," by seeing like a subject, and through housekeeping work—practices that reinforced both the finest traits and the most unsavory biases of each board's membership.

ONE

Everyone's an Expert?
Warrants for Expertise

The Imperative of Consensus

Most of the time board members were not confrontational. Their discussions of research proposals were brief, and their demeanor toward each other was civil. Occasionally, though, they got red-faced. Witness this exchange about reporting suspected child abuse, which unfolded during a late-autumn meeting at Greenly State:

JOHN (FACULTY, ANTHROPOLOGY): But, that's what worries me. You got two choices here. One is you stop doing this research or you set people up so you can catch them, which destroys research, too. And so you get a few people off the street that way. One time around and in the process you end research on this area.

EDWARD (FACULTY, ARCHITECTURE): Oh yeah, John, that's pretty cool. A friend of mine's child was killed /

JOHN: No, I /

EDWARD: Wait, wait, let me finish. You know, a friend of mine's child was killed because he was shook. Because he was shaken. You know, two years old and they found her dead. I don't want to go too far into this, but you know, I loved that person. The research be damned. You know, yeah, it's hard to do research, but if you suspect child abuse then you have to say it.[1]

Consensus among group members is an achievement, not a foregone conclusion. As the exchange between John and Edward makes plain, board members disagreed with their colleagues at times—more placidly, in most cases, but nonetheless pointedly.

IRBs get their authority from administrative law. Open the Code of Federal Regulation, and you will read that the authority to approve, disapprove, or request modification of protocols rests with "the IRB." It is worth noticing who is missing from the federal regulations. There is no mention of individual IRB members, who have no power. This is not to say that individual opinions do not matter. Quite to the contrary: individual members are selected because of their particular knowledge in a specific area. However, because the regulations grant power to the expert body—not to individual experts—it is "the IRB" that has to produce a decision. In other words, administrative law empowers the declarative body to do things that a piece of it—say, Edward—could not accomplish on its own. Like our human bodies, declarative bodies are more than the sum of their parts.[2]

If each board member has an equal claim to expertise, then how do they reach a decision? One option would be to vote, which IRB members do. But IRB votes have an uncanny likeness to each other. Almost without exception, the outcomes that I observed were unanimous, and individual members never voted against the group. To signal their disagreement, board members in a few instances abstained from voting altogether. It was the most damning act of resistance they mustered.

The work of achieving unanimity happened before the vote—when members tuned their individual voices into a chorus that their audience (including researchers, study participants, and the university legal team) could hear as one voice. The appearance of unanimity among members consolidates these individuals into the regulatory actor that is empowered by the law. Consensus creates the impression of a strong, incontrovertible decision and erases the underlying disagreements of individuals who have no authority. IRB documents tend to report a consensual decision because individual members have no authority to act on their own. Thus the pervasiveness of group consensus and the strictly symbolic function of voting are themselves products of the social organization of expert bodies as laid out in federal regulations.[3]

This begs the question: if everyone on the board is an expert with an equally valid claim to his opinion, then how do declarative bodies reach a consensus? One fundamental way in which individual IRB members built a group decision about how rules applied in specific cases was to persuade other members that they had the best backing for their opinion compared to colleagues on the board. The group deliberations that I observed were essentially referenda on who had the most salient knowledge and thus whose advice should be followed.

I use the concept of *warranting* to explain how IRB members reached consensus on group recommendations during their closed-door deliberations. Warrants are reasons or justifications that people give for their views.

In the sections below, I describe three types of warrants that group members used during deliberations. This set of warrants is not exhaustive, to be sure, but I lay out for your inspection three of the most common and persuasive warrants. IRBs also had decision-making habits, that they used when they processed studies that felt familiar and routine (see chapter 2). However, when the proper course of action was either ambiguous or contested, board members reached consensus by deciding whose recommendation was based on the most relevant knowledge, which all members could endorse as the view of "the IRB."

What the warranting process shows at the broadest level is that the actual process of decision making among knowledge experts is quite different from its appearance in formal records. Meeting minutes essentially freeze a moment in time, in particular, the very end of deliberations. The minutes do not allow readers to see what took place beforehand to move all of the elements into position so that "the IRB" could render a decision.[4] Understanding the differences between the process of decision making and the final product of a decision—the letters of judgment sent to researchers, for example—is especially important in studies of governance because IRB members, unlike elected officials, are appointed. Knowledge experts often do not have a clear, tangible set of constituents whose views they are called to articulate and who hold them accountable. Adding to this, declarative bodies often interpret regulations in physical locations that are difficult for most people to access.[5] This chapter gives a chance to step inside one such place.

What Is Warranting?

Members of declarative bodies use warranting as a tool for reaching shared decisions. When warranting their statements, people are implicitly answering the question "Why?" or "On account of what?"[6] When I analyzed my field notes and transcripts of IRB meetings, I coded as warrants the statements that IRB members made to account for their recommendations on how the group should proceed with a study.

Warrants have three distinctive features. First, although they are given verbally, warrants are often implicit in a speaker's language. People tend to use warrants when they are challenged or pushed to justify themselves.[7] Because IRB meetings are organized around making choices, as opposed to talking for its own sake, board members have to account for their views quite frequently.

Second, warrants are context specific, which means that different types of justifications are persuasive in different settings. As sociologist Robert Wuthnow has written, people do not justify their views haphazardly, but "choose ideas that seem legitimate in relation to the *norms* present in their social context." Because of this, warrants "are likely to reflect the norms of which social structure is composed in different contexts."[8] The implication is that the warrants used in IRB meetings tell us how group members understand their setting, by showing us what people are willing to say in a context that many people regard as a bureaucratic social space.

Finally, the success or failure of an individual's warrant is determined by his listeners and whether they accept or reject his justification. This means that an IRB member's warrant is convincing only if fellow board members treat it as such. The study of warrants, as a result, is a pragmatic approach to analyzing group deliberations.

Reaching Consensus

In interviews, many board members described a division of labor among IRB members, both regarding the issues on which they could make judgments and regarding the topics on which colleagues should intervene. In general, they agreed that each member was valued for her or his recommendations in the area of her or his professional training. For example, Dr. Cain, a faculty member who was trained as a physiologist, described himself as being someone who judged, in particular, the quality of the science that investigators proposed. Compared to his colleagues on the Greenly IRB, he explained, "I'm looking at the value of the science whereas I think somebody like Nathan, being an ethicist, he's really looking at more / He's not looking at the science. He's looking at the ethical value or implications of the work." In keeping with this division of labor, Dr. Cain cautioned that community members should not be undervalued, describing them as "some of the most important people there," because they took care of certain review tasks that other IRB members neglected. "They keep the scientists and the medical folks honest [because] their perspective is not to drive or improve the science," he explained, "but is really to protect people. I feel I have that obligation as well, but I think theirs is much more weighted in that direction, so I think they're very important."[9] Like Dr. Cain, other board members described what can be thought of as role-specific norms of participation in IRB meetings during interviews. Still, it is important to note that Dr. Cain felt that he, too, could usefully weigh in on the evaluations that properly belonged to community members.

Community members also saw a close affinity between formally desig-nated roles and appropriate types of recommendations. Reverend Quinn, a community member serving on the Sander IRB, felt that she had brought to the board "a lot of knowledge of what the patient's world was like. . . . In a general sense, I knew what their suffering was like, what their anxieties were." She also felt she had brought "a sense of the values of the commu-nity that I serve, the wider neighborhood, and my church." When I asked whether she could predict the concerns that her colleagues would raise, she tied her colleagues' concerns to their professional training:

> A couple of the doctors I know look at things like blood chemistry, require-ments for pharmaceuticals, and the synergistic effects of things, and I know they're really on the ball with that. And I know that for instance, Kitty, if there's an issue of nursing practice and logistics of how privacy is dealt with in the nursing setting, she's really on top of that stuff. You know, and when she speaks, she seems to be usually right on target with it. In that sense, I think these are people who are very vigilant about their area of expertise. So the whole works together pretty well.[10]

Reverend Quinn's description of board members' complementary roles sounded much like Dr. Cain's account. Also like Dr. Cain, she reserved for herself some latitude to weigh in on issues outside of what she described as her role-specific task. She felt she could judge the quality of research, as she indicated when she lamented that she had seen proposals with "pretty questionable scientific merit be passed through." And by her description, she "cut her teeth" on chemotherapy protocols while serving on other IRBs, so she knew "a lot about the basics of drugs and the things you look for in drug protocols."[11]

IRB members had a shared sense of their individual jobs on the board, as well as the jobs of their colleagues. At the same time, they reserved the right to make recommendations on issues that extended beyond their of-ficial area of specialization. It was not obvious to Reverend Quinn that she should limit herself to discussions about community values, Dr. Cain about scientific merit, Nathan about ethics, or Kitty about nursing practice. There was flexibility in board members' sense of the areas in which they and their colleagues could usefully contribute to deliberations. This flex-ibility was evident in board meetings, in which board members gave their views on topics that they were formally qualified to judge—and on other topics as well.

Claiming Expertise: Three Types of Warrants

The IRB members whom I observed reached consensus by siding with the colleague they thought had the best justification, or warrant, for his or her recommendation. Under conditions of uncertainty or dispute, in other words, board members arrived at decisions by persuading each other with what appeared to them to be good evidence for their views. The warrants that IRB members used took three forms, which I call matters of fact, private experience, and professional experience.

Matters of Fact

IRB members often warranted their views with "objective" findings, often in the form of numbers, such as statistics. Such seemingly objective evidence is authoritative because it is not associated with any one person and instead can take a material form, for example, in a diagram, table, or image.[12] I call warrants based on seemingly disembodied, objective evidence *matters of fact*.

This kind of evidence offers promise for those hopeful about a democratic decision-making process. Scholars have shown how nonspecialists can harness the seemingly universal authority of objective evidence for their own purposes. This is possible, they argue, because objective evidence carries the persuasive power of expert knowledge and yet is accessible outside of expert communities. Sociologists Harry Collins and Robert Evans have pointed out, for example, that today the Internet provides a way for people without formal training to access information traditionally sequestered among experts in a given field. They use the term "primary source knowledge" to describe information that comes from credentialed experts but is widely available to people without formal training in the field. The process through which nonspecialists make effective use of certified knowledge has been cast as a positive move toward the democratization of decision making about science.[13]

What I mean to designate by matters of fact is the kind of knowledge that is shared but comes from specialists: the information that one could learn by studying academic books, reading scholarly journals, or hearing lectures in a given field. This feature of matters of fact made it possible for community members, such as Reverend Quinn, to use statistics to warrant their views. An example of this happened when board members reevaluated a previously approved vaccine trial because the investigator had reported a Serious Adverse Event. (The U.S. Food and Drug Administration requires that researchers report to their IRB when a study participant unexpectedly experiences a problem, which may or may not have been caused by the studies.) A woman enrolled in the vaccine trial had gotten pregnant (against study protocol) and then had a miscarriage. The issue the board was considering was whether to make the investigator change the protocol so that all women enrolled in the study had to use a semipermanent form of birth control, such as a hormone injection, rather than a barrier method, such as diaphragms and condoms.

Reverend Quinn argued against more stringent birth-control requirements for women and warranted her opinion using a matter of fact:

REVEREND QUINN: Condoms are very effective. They fail in [5 to 15 percent of cases /
OWEN (EMERITUS, PHARMACOLOGY): If used!]
REVEREND QUINN: If used *incorrectly*. This patient / This subject reports that she used condoms and had a failure. It happens. It happens. And so, I wouldn't want to raise the bar and say it's not an effective enough birth control. I think (it's fine).[14]

As I coded my field notes and meeting transcripts, I looked, in particular, for moments when IRB members asserted an opinion, and I then tracked how IRB members linked their opinions to accounts of why they held that view. In the exchange about the Serious Adverse Event, Reverend Quinn offered her recommendation: the study should not change because condoms are effective. Then she substantiated it with a warrant: condom failure rates. It is not important whether the evidence that Reverend Quinn used is strictly accurate. What is important is the type of evidence she used—in this case, disembodied, seemingly objective quantitative measures, or matters of fact. The type of evidence she used is important to note because in the end the board acted on the view of Reverend Quinn, whose role on the board, by her own description, was to articulate the sensibilities of research subjects, not to weigh in on birth control statistics. Board members did not require the investigator to make women on the protocol use a semipermanent form of birth control.

Another example comes from Adams Medical IRB. Immediately after a board meeting, I walked with Kimberly, a pediatrician on faculty, to her office. I asked her what she made of a rough discussion the group had worked through during the earlier meeting. Perched in her office chair from behind a desk stacked with papers, she looked as if she existed on a smaller scale than her office furniture. She was young, too, compared with the other physicians on the board, and had photos of a toddler in view. Either because of or despite these signs of femininity, she was reliably assertive in IRB meetings. During the interview, I asked Kimberly why she had urged board members to approve without modifications a hotly contested study that some of her colleagues had strongly resisted. Here is how she explained her position: "I mean, there were recent articles in the *New England Journal* that [said] the chance of actually having major toxicity from the trial is less than 5 percent and toxic death is less than 1 percent, like .5 percent. And the chances of getting, having clinical benefit, true response, is about 10 percent. And stabilization of disease was like 30 to 40 percent. So, actually the chances are not so bad in that stage in disease, that you will get benefits."[15] Kimberly immediately drew on matters of fact to justify her opinion: response rates from a premier medical journal. Interestingly, she continued: "There are certain people that I think make judgments based on sort of visceral feelings about things. And then there are other people that will listen to evidence-based arguments. And I'm probably a mix of both. I have definite / I come to the table with definite visceral responses to things. . . . But, in the end if you can give me a good scientific basis, that's what's going to sway me the most either way."[16]

Kimberly emphasized the importance of matters of fact, or what she called "evidence-based arguments," in describing what she considered persuasive evidence from her colleagues. Her term played on the language of evidence-based medicine, which is a relatively recent and somewhat contested move in health care toward using outcome data, not only clinical judgment, in diagnosis and therapy. But Kimberly also described a second kind of warrant that IRB members used—and which she acknowledged using—based on what she described as "visceral responses."

Private Experience

During IRB meetings, other board members, like Kimberly, justified their recommendations not only with matters of fact but also with reference to their children's fears, their parents' illnesses, or other aspects of what I call *private experience*. What this type of justification lacked in clear logic it often made up for in force of conviction: IRB members' private experiences were extremely emotional warrants. They also constituted a form of common knowledge.[17] Although IRB members were speaking about their own firsthand experiences, all members could warrant their recommendations based on their own knowledge as a parent, child, neighbor, teacher, former student—or any number of roles they used to define their lives.

The exchange at Greenly State recounted at the beginning of this chapter was part of a review of a study on how parents discipline their children. By state law, investigators have to report children whom they suspect may have been abused, a provision that makes research on parenting practices quite delicate. In this case, the investigator planned to ask mothers and fathers to report, in detail, how they punished their children. The investigator made it clear when she spoke with the board that there were no circumstances in which her team would report parents to legal authorities as possible child abusers. Many board members were ambivalent about the study. On the one hand, it seemed to them that at some point the investigator would have to report abuse to stay within the bounds of state law.[18] On the other hand, board members agreed with the investigator that her otherwise very useful and important data would be invalidated ("shaped" or "sanitized") if she trumpeted to parents in advance that she might report them for child abuse. After the investigator left, board members brainstormed ways in which the investigator could collect less detailed data so that she would not be able to even suspect child abuse while still collecting some data on disciplining practices, for example, by changing questions about frequency of hitting children with different items (hand, belt, brush, etc.) into dichotomous variables (e.g., whether parents ever hit their child with a belt). The board was trying to decide how explicit the investigator needed to be. After an extended discussion, John, a cultural anthropologist on faculty at Greenly, lamented what he saw as the board's options—or at least started to lament before getting interrupted by Edward's forceful recommendation backed by reference to a private experience: the death of a friend's child (see page 21).

Each board member, regardless of her or his field of expertise, could tie recommendations to intimate experiences. Like Edward, board members presented their views as part of their personal narrative—the stories that gave their lives texture and feeling. Knowledge experts considered insights drawn from experiences beyond their professional lives to be relevant for evaluating research protocols. And since IRBs are oriented toward mitigating worst-case scenarios, rather than managing "typical," "average," or "common" scenarios, anomalous but vividly or passionately relayed stories were taken to be, if not persuasive, at least difficult to argue against.

In this case, the board did not merely require that the investigator change his measures or report abuse; instead, impassioned personal testimony like that of Edward encouraged members to seek a higher level of scrutiny for the project. The IRB tabled the decision and referred the protocol to university legal offices. After several months with no decision, the investigator abandoned her research plan and withdrew the project from consideration.

Board members used private experience in disputes with each other, but also in disagreements between themselves and investigators who submitted protocols for review. During another review, the IRB administrator at Greenly, Nancy, used a warrant based on her private experience to justify her view that the IRB should make an investigator change the intervention he planned to use in a child psychology study. The investigator was at the meeting, and he described his intervention as "a mild non-traumatic stress," which was essential to examine children's physiological responses to stress, such as how their hormone levels change. Earlier in this meeting, Nancy had lectured the investigator that the intervention would be much more stressful for children than he imagined. He responded:

INVESTIGATOR: For myself, clinically, it's hard for me to imagine that this would be traumatic. But others [could argue /
NANCY (IRB ADMINISTRATOR): For my eight year old] grandson, this would be hideously traumatic.
NATHAN (FACULTY, PHILOSOPHY): Yeah.[19]

The investigator was silenced. As this interaction suggests, when members articulated their recommendations in terms of their private experiences, it was difficult for others to argue against what they claimed to know—to contradict their lived experiences. The discussion also shows the beginning of a consensus built around Nancy's opinion that the investigator should not be allowed to do the stress intervention as planned. The ethicist who agreed with Nancy here went on to explain that, having recently become a father, he seconded Nancy's view. Eventually all of the board members came to side with Nancy's recommendation, based on her private experiences, rather than the view of the investigator, based on his clinical experience.

Nancy's opinion helped to shift the research design of this study. One curious feature of the regulatory structure of IRBs is that in the legal imagination, official board members would be expected to affect researchers' plans as knowledge experts. In the regulations, people like Nancy—that is to say, IRB administrators—are phantoms. Their presence is implicit in the requirement that IRBs keep careful records and produce documents sent to researchers. Their involvement in discussions as a feeling, attentive person is not anticipated in the regulations. And the legitimacy of their claims in deliberations has not been fully acknowledged and debated.

Professional Experience

IRB members also recommended changes to protocols by tying their advice to their special experiences as knowledge producers. I call this third kind of warrant *professional experience*. The cultural authority of knowledge-producing professions—the sciences, medicine, and the humanities, for example—depends on the notion that practitioners acquire unique and valuable skills through their training and professional experience. These experiences, moreover, are generally thought to translate into rare abilities to judge the quality, veracity, or ethics of knowledge outside of research settings. This is why experts are often allowed to carry the authority they have derived from one setting to another, for example, from the bench to the bedside, the lab to the courtroom, the field to the review panel, and the armchair to the lectern.

The power of professional experience was apparent in one case in which members of the Sander State IRB were reviewing a study on arthritis in elderly people. The investigators were recruiting arthritic men via courses offered through the National Arthritis Foundation. In other studies, investigators had collected a good deal of information about this population, and the investigator under review hoped to tap these existing data. The primary IRB reviewer, Dr. Endicott, had given the proposal a positive review, and the study seemed poised to sail through to full-board approval. Right before the vote for approval, however, another board member, an exercise physiologist named Ulrich, argued for changes to the protocol that would seriously decrease study enrollment. Another board member, Denise, worked hard to counter Ulrich's recommendations. Ultimately, Denise was not successful in persuading her colleagues of her opinion because Ulrich anchored his opinion to his professional experience as an exercise physiologist.

Here is how it unfolded. Poised for the vote, the warranting contest began when Ulrich urged IRB members to require an additional screening questionnaire for study participants:

ULRICH (EXERCISE PHYSIOLOGIST): With reference to my background, there's a health questionnaire (used in) other studies, and it does a good job of referring to how [people] feel (at different levels of exertion).[20]

Importantly, Ulrich specifically linked his opinion to what he called his professional "background." Then he continued by recounting one of his own experiences as a researcher before the time when questionnaires were widely used to screen for appropriate research participants:

ULRICH (CONTINUING): I'll give you an example: my first year here in 1992, we had someone on a treadmill who had a spinal cord injury with support, and the student came up and said "excuse me, but I don't think we should be testing this subject. He has an aortic aneurism."
GROUP: *h h h*[21]

The board members' laughter suggests how untoward Ulrich's anecdote sounded: he had encouraged a person with a serious heart condition to exercise. But Denise resisted changing the study when Ulrich again made his specific request to add an additional screening questionnaire:

ULRICH: I would suggest a questionnaire that has been approved by the IRB in a previous study that deals with current medical history that is associated with cardiac patients, or physiological stress.
DENISE (NURSING FACULTY): But this isn't a physiologic stress test, is it, Ulrich? I mean
ULRICH: When you get up to 130 beats a minute, sixty-five years old. You take 220 minus 65, divide that [by 130 and you get, the person's a 70 or 80 percent of predicted maximum heart rate, then / You know, we have our guidelines.
DENISE: Yeah, I know. Um hum. Sure. Sure.]
BETH (HISTORIAN): It sounds like a prudent thing to do.
GROUP: (Yeah, it's prudent).[22]

Note here that the board members—including Denise—started to align themselves with Ulrich. This, again, was the beginning of a consensus. Denise persisted, explaining what was at stake in a seemingly minor change to a protocol, telling board members, "You run the risk in this population, especially if [the investigator] is recruiting from senior centers, of eliminating lots of people who would not necessarily have an issue." Then, to warrant her competing viewpoint, she tied her opinion to professional experience of her own. Other IRB members, however, rejected her claim to relevant professional experience:

DENISE: I'm trying to think back to the senior project I worked on. There was an exercise piece to that, and I don't believe we had any exclusion. They were people that were community residing and already in exercise programs, it seems to me, just as this one is.

ELIZABETH (IRB ADMINISTRATOR): That was really very low level exercise.

KITTY (NURSING FACULTY): Didn't use treadmills. They didn't use bicycles.[23]

In the end, Ulrich's warrant based on his professional experience swayed members. Most influentially, Ulrich had persuaded Dr. Endicott, the main IRB member charged with presenting this study to the board. Although Denise made her case yet again, it was to no avail:

DENISE: Again, I think that these are people that have been exercising anyway. I'm not supportive of the idea of having exclusions / It just worries me a bit that it gets so tight that there may not be a population (left to study). With this age group that's really possible.

MADELINE (FACULTY MEMBER AND IRB CHAIR): Dr. Endicott?

DR. ENDICOTT (NONFACULTY GENERAL PRACTITIONER): I agree with Ulrich. I think that's an excellent idea to include that health questionnaire that this IRB already approved several years ago for the physical therapy department to put on here.

As this discussion showed, IRB members tended to defer to recommendations of the member who articulated experiences as a knowledge producer in a field that was most similar to the field of the investigator. In some instances, this board member recommended harsher restrictions on the investigator's work based on his own experience, and at other times he urged the group to loosen constraints. Regardless of the direction of change, though, it was the similarity of the expert's professional experience that appeared compelling, rather than the relative authority of an expert's academic discipline or medical specialty.[24]

In their native settings, scholars and scientists record their sensory perceptions—the things they see, hear, and feel—as numbers, words, and images because it allows them more easily to communicate and advocate for resources from the government. At root, however, scientists' truth claims are based on tacit, embodied skills, which are eventually translated into objective-seeming measurements. Scholars who study "knowledge production"—that is to say, the processes through which scientists claim to discover facts of nature—have shown that becoming an expert requires learning how to "see" or to "read" potential evidence according to the conventions of one's scientific community. These are skills that knowledge workers have to develop through apprenticeship and physical practice. A good example of this point is the finding that, despite the inclusion of technologies in scientific work, researchers cannot reproduce the outcomes of a colleague's experiment if they have not spent time in the same location together, teaching and learning the physical skills needed to run the equipment and the experiment. The uninitiated have to learn from established practitioners how to create and recognize would-be evidence. In its most carnal form, embodied knowledge is based on the senses, especially on sight and touch, in the sciences.[25]

The Triumph of Professional Experience?

IRB members built a group consensus out of their individual claims to knowledge about the matter at hand. To do so, board members gave recommendations and then warranted their views in one of three ways: by articulating matters of fact, private experience, or professional experience. This framework begs the following question: when different warrants are pitted against each other, which one do board members take to be most persuasive? There is no way to answer this question numerically. For some questions, word counts and checked boxes cannot capture the fullness or fluidity of interactions. That is the strength of observational research—but also its limit. With this caveat in mind, I will describe and explain how board members treated their colleagues' professional experiences as most persuasive in the meetings I watched, and illustrate this with one final example.

The case comes from a protocol review at Greenly State. For this study, a well-funded social psychologist on faculty planned an emotions-management course at the university's laboratory school. The investigator's aim was to assess whether children would better temper their frustrations and enthusiasms after they had taken an expert-designed behavior-training course. To control for any effects that the children's family background might have on their behavior, the parents who consented and the children who assented would be given several psychological tests via interviews. Board members' initial views were positive.

But after the three preliminary reviewers made their points—they were a physiologist, a philosopher, and a pastor—another board member, a psychologist named Kevin, interjected an opinion. He urged board members to require what he considered to be a very substantial change to the study, one that would restrict enrollment. Kevin said the investigator should specifically state in the consent form that the research team would test the parents' and children's IQs and would keep the scores on file (without linked identifying information). To justify his view that the study should be changed, Kevin drew from his professional experience with the measure that the investigator intended to use. Kevin described the investigator as "world famous."

He asserted, "She is Ms. Human Emotions in kids. Okay. She's (built up) grad students for years and she's got these projects." Kevin continued: "But I mean to tell you, the Bailey, I helped develop it, okay. That's an IQ test. That's not mentioned in there. I mean we're quibbling about a vocabulary measure. But that's an IQ test! That's proxy for IQ. I'm kind of, ahh / You know, if I were to read this letter [addressed to the parents] and knowing what I know about assessment: they're not lining up at all. Not at all."[26]

As in many reviews, there was more than one recommendation, which depended on different warrants, about how best to proceed. In this case, Nancy, the IRB administrator, said she felt that the investigator should not have to modify the study because she was a well-known, diligent researcher who had the best interest of the children in mind. How did she know? Because of her own experiences seeing her children and grandchildren through this lab school. As she put it, "I know from previous experience with a lot of this she doesn't want to frighten people."[27]

Recall that Nancy had warranted her opinions successfully in other cases by invoking her private experiences. Previously we heard her persuade board members to accept her recommendation using knowledge she derived from her experience as a grandmother. In this instance, however, Nancy's private experiences butted up against Kevin's professional experiences. Kevin eventually addressed Nancy's counterpoint directly, saying to her, "Well, you don't want to frighten people because people start saying no. And *h*. That's hard though. *h*."

Throughout the discussion, IRB members aligned behind Kevin. In reaction, board members said, for example, "I think that's right," and "Yes, I can see your point." One light-hearted exchange revealed board members' deference to Kevin's specialist knowledge. The board chair got a laugh from board members by exclaiming to Kevin, "Bailey doesn't mean anything to anybody except you."[28]

In the end, board members were persuaded by Kevin's view, and all of the debate—the complexities, disagreements, and uncertainties between Nancy and Kevin—were smoothed over when "the IRB" rendered its judgment. The letter to the investigator stated that "the Board" requested that the investigator include in the consent form "a brief description, in lay language, of each of the measures" that researchers would be taking of parents and children. (I return in chapter 3 to this case and the work of inventing "the IRB" through documents).

As Kevin's success also shows, all warrants are not equal. Warrants based on professional experience were most persuasive in the IRB meetings I observed because they were based on members' specialist knowledge, making these warrants a rare commodity. Professional warrants are also based on embodied, firsthand knowledge, which renders them very difficult to challenge on their own terms.

The IRB members who often swayed decisions most systematically in board meetings were those who justified their recommendations with a claim to research experience relevant to the case at hand, even if the study came from outside of the board member's discipline. IRB members recounted their research experiences as a means, in the absence of other routines for establishing credibility, to persuade colleagues that their advice was valid and worth following. But warrants based on professional experience were not available to all IRB members. Only members who claimed training as a relevant specialist could use this apparently convincing form of justification. In short, warrants are not equally persuasive, nor are they equally available to board members.

Conclusion: Claiming Authority

The ways in which IRB members warranted their views cut two ways. They portrayed the knowledge on which their recommendations were based as either experiential or objective and as either part of the wider knowledge network or part of their particular life story. Surprisingly, the full range of IRB members, from pediatricians to administrators, justified their recommendations based on experiences in their private lives. Historian Steven Shapin has argued that experts at times offer accounts of their own lives quite strategically (though not necessarily reflexively) in an effort to persuade clients that their professional advice is worth following.[29]

When the textured lives of colorful characters were arranged around the conference table, the IRB took on a vital form that federal regulations empowered and animated—but perhaps in surprising ways. Everyone sitting around the table, for example, drew on private experiences to warrant recommendations regardless of the person's official evaluative task as a board member. Mark Brown points out in his study of government advisory committees, "The knowledge of most experts is so specialized that they are effectively lay people with regard to issues beyond their immediate area of expertise."[30] Yet IRB members' broad use—and the rhetorical usefulness—of private experiences highlights the fact that expert members did not finely differentiate the reasons on which they based their assessments of researchers' studies. It is sometimes assumed that nonexperts' private experiences are a resource unique to them—which they might use persuasively if only they were included in deliberations. This imagined gap between what citizens or community members know that knowledge experts do not articulate is a by-product of a democratic illusion. One might wish that there could be a pure representative of the common good or of the conceptual populations to be protected—children, women, prisoners—but of course an ideal, composite representative exists in theory only. This raises practical questions about who should have legitimate authority to participate in decisions, and on what grounds. IRB members' ability to transcend narrow evaluative tasks could be seen in either a positive or a negative light. Should regulators hand muzzles or bullhorns to people who are authorized based on their expertise to participate in decisions when they use their private experiences to reach decisions?[31] The same might be asked of IRB administrators. Just because they are not named in regulations as participants, should they not be able to register opinions?

In unexpected ways, the issue of who gets authorized to sit around the table has a remarkable effect on the decision-making process. First, I saw that experts' firsthand experience with particular research methods shaped conversations more than members' affiliation with one academic discipline or topic of specialty affected discussion. Group members had a harder time challenging their colleagues with reasons drawn from outside of conventional professional practices. By deferring to a member's professional experience—as opposed to personal stories or "evidence-based" knowledge—structures of authority are stabilized through group deliberation. That said, it might also be worthwhile to reenvision investigators as important participants in discussions because their trained experience might offer a firm point of reference. Second, the powerful effect of board members' personal experiences on decisions shows that the people who feature in the lives of IRB members outside of the office deeply inform how they evaluate research when they come into the conference room. It is an open question whether experts' personal experiences—not the knowledge that brought them into the board room in the first place—are a legitimate basis for decisions. What is clear is that board members' networks of friends, neighbors, and relatives guide the evaluation process.

Still, the fact that everyone used private experiences to flesh out the pleasures and pains of research may reveal as much about the individuals as about how to conceptualize the setting of bureaucracy behind closed doors. A good part of government decision making happens in restricted settings that most people cannot access. Many questions raised about declarative bodies as a tool of government have gone unanswered precisely because administrative groups work outside of public view. Witness not only IRBs but the expert bodies within federal agencies such as the Environmental

Protection Agency, the Office of Research Integrity, the Food and Drug Administration, and the Federal Reserve.[32]

The ways in which experts interpret rules is contingent upon their immediate audience, and specifically upon whether representatives of "the public," such as citizens and their proxies (e.g., legislators) are in the audience. If IRB meetings are anything to go by, decision makers are persuaded by different forms of evidence for administrative choices made behind closed doors than in decisions made publicly, with doors flung open, TV cameras rolling, and full transcripts available. In settings where knowledge experts make decisions with little public record, I would anticipate that firsthand, experiential, embodied knowledge would be persuasive, as it was in IRBs that I observed. When decisions are translated outside of these cloistered settings for public consumption, the justifications on which group members make decisions may either drop away entirely or be scrubbed clean of personal idiosyncrasy (that is to say, illegitimacy). The techniques of persuasion that are most effective among experts in "restricted settings," such as IRB meetings, have been shown to be ineffectual and often corrosive for experts who have been called to account for their views in "open settings," for example in congressional hearings, legislative debates, and legal trials.[33] The workings of IRBs would suggest that, for better or worse, settings with high public exposure will generate more warrants based on objective evidence. Conversely, in settings that have low public exposure or accountability, decision makers will rely more heavily on warrants based on subjective evidence.

Expert bodies, that is to say, would produce different decisions not only if different speakers were present in deliberations, but also if there were a different audience for their deliberations. Adding listeners would fundamentally change the setting of decision making from a de facto private setting to a more public setting. Posting transcripts of deliberations online, for example, could create a radically different audience for decision makers and, more importantly, would likely give decision makers a different imagined audience: namely, any member of the computer-savvy public, rather than only their colleagues sitting across the conference table. Changing the audience for the decision-making process is key to changing the outcomes of actual decisions, because decision makers' sense of their listeners would appear to alter their willingness to endorse recommendations based on personal knowledge rather than matters of fact. What I am advocating, then, is a return to the ideas of Basil Bernstein, who championed comparative studies of open and restricted settings because, he theorized, conventions of appropriate language use allow different ideas and generalizations to emerge in different settings.[34] It is a provocative claim that remains an open question.

To return to the question for this chapter: Is everyone equally an expert in IRB meetings? In theory, the answer is yes. In practice, however, the answer is no. This dual answer points to the promise and the peril of deliberative decision making. Since the 1960s governments have relied increasingly on groups of experts to enact regulations, which give abstract rules their concrete meaning in the lives of citizens. Cordoned off from traditional avenues of public oversight, declarative bodies have been imagined as democratic by virtue of their design. Each member is expert in his field; each member is equally valuable.

The puzzle is how expert bodies reach decisions without any formal hierarchy.[35] The IRBs I observed demonstrated that their decisions were in part the product of a warranting process, through which members decided who had the most persuasive claim to knowledge on the matter at hand. The type of evidence that a speaker used to justify her recommendation worked to persuade or dissuade listeners of the merit of her view and, consequently, of the wisdom of harnessing the group's authority to the recommendation. Thus, "good" recommendations are, by my account, social achievements and not reflections of the inherent qualities of the recommendations themselves.

Attention to warrants enriches current efforts to explain group decisions. First, it offers a fuller explanation of group decision making (and its disparities) by emphasizing how language strategies can build or break down consensus during the course of deliberations. Other factors certainly affect the decision-making process. The relationships that people build outside of meetings help to explain how groups achieve consensus in the official moment of deliberation.[36] It is also clear that decision outcomes are patterned on group members' personal traits, including gender. But attention to warrants reveals what it is about individuals' traits that make some members appear to have a knack for affecting decisions—namely, that the *types* of justifications that individuals have at their disposal are a consequence of their past opportunities and experiences.

TWO

Local Precedents

Dissonant Decisions

Men who have been arrested and incarcerated have a significantly harder time getting a job than men with no criminal record. But the situation is especially difficult for black men. If a black man has been in prison, he is less than half as likely to be considered for a job than an ex-offender whose skin color happens to be white.[1]

This is an important research finding. It is also a good example of how our notions of justice and our perceptions of public policies often change as researchers in medicine and the social sciences learn new things about individuals and social groups. Yet despite potential positive outcomes of this research, one could argue that the research methods were deceptive and unfair to the people being studied. The research involved sending fake job candidates—one white man and one black man—to apply in person for jobs advertised in a local newspaper. The men filled out the applications in identical ways. On some applications they said they had been convicted of a crime; on other applications they said they had a clean record. They made sure each employer got a good look at them. Then they waited for a phone call. The employers were under study, but they had never agreed to be the focus of the researcher's gaze, and they wasted time and money screening bogus applicants.

Was it worth it? I would say yes, but others would disagree. Could it have been made a bit more fair to employers, who, after all, were not multibillion-dollar corporations but businesses trying to make ends meet in Milwaukee? When I asked this question to IRB chairs from large universities across the United States, almost all thought their board would have required changes to the study, if they had let it go ahead at all. I then asked, "How would the researcher need to change the study?" Each answer to this question was as distinctive as the place where the board was located.

It is a puzzle—and a persistent problem for investigators—that different IRBs never seem to agree on how research should be conducted. It is a consequence of the unintuitive design of our current decentralized review system, in which there are as many IRBs as there are sites hosting research. This causes a serious practical problem for many researchers who face competing and sometimes contradictory judgments from several boards about how a single study needs to be modified before it can be approved. In recent years, the number of multisite studies that draw human subjects from several locations has been on the rise, and each institution has its own IRB that must approve the research.[2] Imagine a clinical trial that recruits patients through hospitals across the United States because the disease under study is rare or because the trial requires thousands of volunteers. In these instances, several IRBs have jurisdiction over how the study is carried out. But regardless of location, all board members are following the same set of regulations. Then why do boards come up with different answers?

What Would You Do?

I asked the chairs of IRBs from eighteen major research universities from across the country how their boards would handle a study like the one on race-based hiring discrimination against ex-offenders.[3] The IRB chairs gave very different answers, but they also gave hints as to why IRBs apply the same set of regulations to the same proposals in different ways. Their responses suggest a way to rethink how expert bodies evaluate research and help to explain why IRBs, in particular, arrive at different decisions about the same study.

As the board chairs thought through and talked about the protocol, they did one of two things. Some chairs tried to apply the general human-subjects regulations to this specific case, remarking, for example, that they would "go to the guide book, and look and see what it says about that."[4] One chair stated that she would consult the regulations and "follow the guidelines for research that governs deception."[5] These board members were looking at the proposal with fresh eyes and were inclined to translate general rules so that they could be applied to this specific case, as if for the first time.

Other board chairs saw problems and proposed modifications to the protocol because they recognized it as similar to a memorable study or problem that they had already seen, debated, and resolved. That is to say, they tried to work from an exemplary case to this specific case. Among different communities of researchers, IRBs naturally end up reviewing different protocols, and so each board has its own set of exemplary cases that guide their evaluations of subsequent studies. For the board chairs whom I interviewed, this meant that the standard protocol that I gave them represented widely divergent concerns, based on the particular set of protocols they had reviewed and decisions they had made in the past.

Here was the question: What would your IRB do in this situation?

> Your committee receives a proposal that requests approval for a field experiment. The researcher wants to learn whether employers discriminate against job candidates who are black in comparison to job candidates who are white. The experiment involves black men and white men who are confederates of the researcher and who fill out job applications, preferably in front of the employer, at places where blue-collar jobs have been advertised. The researcher's confederates are trained in advance to behave as similarly as possible. They leave a phone number on the job application. The researcher's dependent variable is whether the confederate gets a call about the job from the potential employer.[6]

It is not apparent from this vignette when or how the researcher might ask employers' consent to include them in the study. Today, informed consent is widely considered to be the foundation of human-subjects protections (though this seemingly intuitive marker of good ethics took on its current shape very recently; see chapter 5). That said, federal regulations do allow IRBs to waive consent for an investigator doing some types of research if the study cannot be carried out in any other way and if the study poses risks that are no greater than what the research subject would experience in his everyday life.[7]

IRB chairs' responses to this protocol ranged widely. "Would we approve it? Yes," one chair replied decisively, "I think this is a pretty cut and dried scenario to tell you the truth."[8] Others were much more ambivalent. "I suspect that this is not something that would go through," another concluded, "This would be extremely problematic."[9]

Although the IRB chairs gave different answers to the question of how the protocol should be handled, they gave compelling justifications for why their board would make a given decision. They did this by recognizing the protocol as an example of a type of research that their board systematically managed in a certain way, as one chair indicated when she immediately spoke of the study in the plural. She remarked, "We are very sympathetic to these," by which she meant studies like an analysis of school quality that her board had approved because it was of "social value" even through it involved deception. "Basically, we're inclined to approve them."[10]

The studies that boards had reviewed in the past not only shaped remedies to ethical concerns but also guided the problems that board chairs read into the protocol in the first place. The chair who had described this study as "extremely problematic," for example, identified risks in the protocol beyond those recognized by most chairs. Like others, she argued that there were serious legal risks to the employers being studied if the investigator breached confidentiality and it became known publicly that certain employers were discriminating against job candidates. From her perspective, however, there were additional risks. She identified the protocol as analogous to research that her committee had previously considered that put at risk not only subjects, but investigators and the university as well. "I can imagine if you're someone accused of discrimination, you're going to pursue this and [possibly even] sue the researcher. So one thing that we're careful about—We have people who are doing research studies on sex workers, say, or transgender people, who are often in high-risk areas and environments carrying out their research. And we're as concerned about the safety of the researchers as the subjects in this case." Thus she felt that her board would see the proposed study as posing risks to the researcher as well as to the subjects, even if those risks were legal rather than physical. She continued, "We'd want to make sure that the person doing this research was protected as well."[11] The added protection that her board would require before approving the protocol might include a federal certificate of confidentiality for the study, which only one other IRB chair proposed.

The primary concern for a different IRB chair was the validity of the research. "We had a study where they were basically doing something very similar to this except they were going to have policemen come by to see if they actually stopped to talk to people or not, depending on whether they were African American or not." His board felt that the study, as originally proposed, was not well designed. "The problem is," he explained, "you might find out about that one [policeman], but if you want to generalize from this whole study that you're doing [to say] that the police department is this way, the problem is that you didn't actually have all possible policemen actually do this." This experience with problems of study design in field research had implications for the standard protocol I gave him: "In this particular case, you're really only studying a small number of people. . . . There are a lot of study protocol things that would have to be there for this to be considered a valid piece of research."[12]

Most board chairs identified informed consent as a concern, but they diverged dramatically on what modifications they would require. One IRB chair saw prior consent as not only possible, but valuable in this protocol because it would both protect the subjects and serve as the ethical linchpin that would allow the research to meet federal regulations without compromising the study design. This was possible in his view because his board had developed an almost formulaic way in which it required investigators to get subjects' consent in deception studies. "We'll say you can describe things in a general way and not be specific, like 'We have a study of attitudes.' And you make them think it's about the passage they're reading but it's actually the pictures that accompany the passage and so on. We'd have real problems with your walking in on somebody and not even making them a willing subject of research."[13] This meant that his board would not approve the study "as it stands" because the employers would not know they are being researched, but if the research got "some kind of prior consent by the party," then his board would likely approve it. He knew from experience that this was entirely possible.

An anthropologist serving as her IRB's chair saw the lack of informed consent as a problem for the study, and yet, try as she might, she could not call to mind a similar study to guide her. Her response is revealing: "Here's some really important research, but my god, there's no consent here. And if there were consent, it wouldn't be worth anything." She concluded, "I just don't see how we could approve that," and then, turning the question to me, asked, "Do you?"[14]

She was one of several board chairs who asked me not what the "right" answer was to the standard protocol, but, in the words of another chair, "How have other people been responding?"[15] When the protocol did not conjure up an exemplary study or problem that the board had previously settled, chairs at times turned to the regulations for guidance, but they also tried to learn about other boards' decisions for a precedent they might adopt. (Tellingly, members of the boards that I observed also asked me how the other boards that I studied handled a problem that they were facing for the first time.) I described to the anthropologist the response of an IRB chair on the East Coast who had proposed that deception "is not necessary in this case." She had recommended telling subjects during the recruitment and consent that sometime in the next year, an imposter job seeker would fill out an employment application. She had found that this strategy had worked well in her own research on discrimination in health care because "[if] you let enough time lapse . . . [subjects] return to their normal behavior."[16]

Hearing this solution, the anthropologist changed her answer, agreeing with delight, "I think that's reasonable."[17]

In the end, all but one chair reported that they could envision a scenario in which the board would allow an investigator to conduct this study if he made certain changes and concessions. However, the chairs diverged on whether they turned to the "rule book" or drew on a resonant past experience. They also diverged in their interpretations of the problems with the study and the modifications that they requested. Because of their unique caseloads prior to my interview, IRB chairs had different views about what risks the standard protocol entailed, who would be at risk, and what the severity of the risk would be. This previous experience guided them toward distinctive decisions about whether consent could be waived, whether investigators could get consent without invalidating their data, and whether debriefing should be mandatory or prohibited as a source of harm in its own right.

Explaining Dissonance

Surveys agree: when different boards are presented with the same standard protocol to review, the boards will unfailingly arrive at different judgments about how the protocol needs to be changed before they will approve it. Survey results, however, have fallen short in explaining why this happens. Authors of these studies tend to view variable decisions as the product of uneven resources across boards. They suggest that with larger staffs, more time, and better training, all boards would arrive at the "correct" decision about a protocol. Locating the source of uneven decisions in uneven material resources does have some merit, and it is certainly a compelling explanation when looking at the externally measurable features of IRBs, such as budgets and decision outcomes. These are only partial explanations, though. Even if IRBs had comparable amounts of funding and staff time at their disposal, they still would not produce wholly consistent decisions.

This is because the differences between IRBs rest not only with their material resources, but with their conceptual resources.[18] The application of general rules to specific cases is always an act of interpretation, since concepts like risk are not inherently meaningful. Recall that to establish working definitions of abstract regulatory terms, IRB members warranted their views about the right course of action when a proposed study presented them with a new puzzle (chapter 1). Another tool IRBs used to reach decisions, the current chapter shows, is to invent the perception of familiar cases. Expert bodies can ease the burden of review by dealing with their workload in a routine way: speedily, consistently, flatly. Routines have to be established, however. They emerge through practice over the course of time.

Each board imprints the studies they review with their common knowledge and experiences as a group. Boards treat many reviews as routine encounters with familiar cases that they know how to handle. This sense of recognition of new studies that, strictly speaking, board members have never seen before marks the importance of board members' shared experiences that serve as the group's common ground. In these circumstances, boards are not working from general rules to specific cases, but from exemplary case to specific case.

I call these exemplary cases *local precedents*. I use this term to describe the past decisions that guide board members' evaluations of subsequent research. By drawing on local precedents, board members can read new protocols as permutations of studies that they have previously debated and settled based on members' warrants. The result is that IRBs tend to make decisions that are locally consistent over time. Whereas board members used individual-level warrants to justify their views to each other, local precedents can be thought of as shared warrants that compel the board as a whole. The important feature of IRBs' local precedents is that they tend to be idiosyncratic to each board but reasonably stable within them, which explains how two well-supported, fully functioning IRBs can arrive at different decisions about the selfsame protocol.

Local precedents can be observed only if IRBs are seen as groups developing over time. This feature of IRBs brings together two insights: first, that small groups develop distinct ways of understanding and acting in the world, and, second, that the timing and order of events structures the paths that people choose to take in the future, a sort of rambling path-dependency.[19] Tying these two threads together, expert bodies have their own histories that shape their distinctive ways of understanding the empirical world.

Local Precedents

After the Sander State IRB discussed an adverse event in a study that they had previously approved, a psychologist on the board, Ken, pithily reflected on the board's new position toward subject recruitment: "Sometimes things have to happen before you know what to do in the future."[20] Ken's observation flags the process in which board members used one evaluation as a stock decision to judge new protocols. Far from applying federal regulations afresh to each new study, they instead identified most new studies as examples of problems they had previously solved. IRB members develop and use local precedents to smooth or speed their future decisions, allowing local boards to make more efficient and internally consistent decisions over time. By the same token, this process is responsible for the variability and inefficiency across IRBs that many critics lament.

In the IRB meeting at Sander State that Ken was reflecting on, board members had been considering investigators' use of what are called opt-out forms in recruiting participants. Investigators can give opt-out forms along with regular consent forms to people invited to participate in a study. If a person does not want to participate, she can send the opt-out form back to the investigator rather than not return the regular consent form. Opt-out forms are generally considered an advance in human-subjects protections because they give people more agency, but many board members have reservations about them because they also force people to respond to a study (if they don't send back a form, either the consent form or the opt-out form, they receive a follow-up call). Views of how investigators should use opt-out forms in their recruitment of research participants varied across the IRBs that I observed.

At Sander, IRB members had always allowed investigators to carry out what seemed to be a common practice: to call potential research subjects on the phone if they did not return a consent form that the investigator had mailed to them. That said, the practice had not passed without remark among board members; they periodically raised questions about whether this aggressive recruitment strategy compromised people's privacy for the sake of higher research enrollment. In their December meeting, for example, the Sander IRB reviewed a study in which the investigator proposed to examine the effectiveness of a behavior-management course for children who showed signs of developing an attention deficit disorder. The investigator planned to have school children carry letters home to their parents introducing the study and asking the parents to return the consent form if they wanted to have their children screened for the disorder and possibly enrolled in the course. If parents did not want to have their children involved in the study, they were instructed not to return the form. However, Nigel, a humanities professor on the board, observed that everyone who did not want to participate in the study would also get a phone call asking whether she had received the information and, again, whether she and her child would like to participate. Nigel pointed out, "It says not to return the form if you're not interested in participating." The investigator assured the board that the research team planned to call just "to make sure" that the person had clearly decided not to participate, but Nigel wondered, "Is this an invasion of privacy?" The investigator suggested that an unreturned consent form might indicate simply that a parent had misplaced the document, not that she was uninterested in the study. With this explanation, the IRB chair moved the discussion onward.[21]

Two months later, at its February meeting, the board was due to renew its approval of a study examining how people with depression managed their condition. The investigators in this study screened tens of thousands of people to find potential volunteers, some of whom were contacted using the records kept on people who had been prescribed antidepressants. A small number of these people complained about the phone call that they received asking whether they wanted to participate in the study. None of the people who complained had received the letter sent to them in advance, introducing the study, along with an opt-out form. The phone call was the next step in the investigators' protocol to pursue potential subjects who had failed to reply either that they were interested or that they were uninterested in participating.

Preempting any IRB decision about whether or how to proceed with the research, the investigators in this study abandoned their strategy of using opt-out forms altogether. They enrolled only people who actively returned consent forms and did not call people who had not sent back their forms. They made this change because the nonconsenting people either would have opted out or they would have been subject to what was now being framed as an invasion of privacy if the investigators called to follow up. The investigators knew that this would reduce the number of subjects they would enroll. They hoped that they would still get enough subjects to run their statistical analyses, perhaps believing that their own conservative solution to the adverse events would be better than remedies that the IRB could require. Assessing the problem and the investigators' response, the IRB agreed that the new plan was the right solution. Furthermore, board members decided, in the words of one member, "We now have a new methodology . . . for similar situations."[22]

It is worth noting that the IRB's "new methodology" emerged to address a practice that they had seen in the past but had never fully considered a problem. This case suggests that complaints from potential recruits and active participants, as well as proposed solutions from investigators, can prompt IRBs to identify and then settle problems that serve as exemplars going forward. The role of investigators in shaping local precedents—which are the solutions that subsequently guide decisions on similar problems—is striking in comparison to investigators' loss of influence over decisions after precedents are set. Investigators can guide IRB decisions, then, but most

effectively during the critical moments when IRBs are settling newly prob-
lematized human-subjects concerns.

Once a local precedent started to crystallize—which was only apparent
when board members applied a one-time decision for the second time to
a new case—board members tended to read subsequent protocols in light
of the past decision. The Greenly IRB, for example, pieced together a local
policy for how investigators can "re-contact" former subjects without their
consent. The philosopher on the board, Nathan, had gently raised this issue
in the past, suggesting to an investigator during the board's April meeting,
"Looking ahead, you might want to do a follow-up study, so you might
want something in the consent to allow you to re-contact them."[23] The conversation started and ended there.

The next month, however, the board was faced with an urgent recontacting issue that proved difficult for them to resolve. An investigator
in child development had planned a new study around the assumption
that she would be allowed to call her former subjects to recruit volunteers.
This would give her a rich data set, because she could merge the new data
with participants' responses from her previous study. Technically, Nathan
argued, this was a breach of an implicit contract with the participants, who
had previously consented to have their contact information used for one
study and had not formally agreed to be identified and sought out again. He
asked the investigator, "How much of a pain would it be to change your recruitment given that you haven't had permission to re-contact?"[24] Recruiting
a new set of subjects, though possible, would severely limit the usefulness
of her proposed study, the investigator replied.

Board members weighed different options. One possibility was to have
the investigator send her former subjects a letter introducing the new study,
before calling them to ask whether they would participate. Another possibility that a board member came up with in his effort to "think creatively"
was to send a letter introducing the study and an opt-out postcard that people could send back if they did not want to get a recruitment phone call.
While board members felt bad that either of these recontacting strategies
would reduce the investigator's enrollment, many also felt that these solutions were less intrusive than unannounced recruiting phone calls. Other
members rolled their eyes at these suggestions.

"I think we're making this a bigger thing than we need to," Edward said.
Donna, from the Sociology Department, agreed: "I don't think that it's the
board's responsibility to protect people from any minor annoyance. I think
that we (should) balance risk against (benefit), and I think that the risk is so
minute in this instance that I would say (you should just contact people).

For the future, perhaps, (include language asking whether you can) contact them in the future." Nathan agreed that the annoyance of being recontacted would be "trivial" and that his colleagues had suggested sensible alternatives. Nonetheless, Nathan said, the problem remained that the IRB was condoning the investigator's breach of contract, and he reminded board members, "We haven't answered the first question, which is whether we're okay with breaching these obligations in the first place, or whether there's any way of making this not a breach of those obligations." Adding to the group's ambivalence, the board chair informed other members that allowing this to proceed could cause trouble in the research office, reporting, "We do get phone calls from people who do not want to be called again. I can guarantee you, we get those. . . . They're very real."[25]

In the end, board members agreed that the investigator would be allowed to break the letter of the law. In the words of the IRB chair, "If there is a problem, this is where we'd have to say to the government, 'Sorry, we've done something incorrectly,' and get our hand slapped." At the same time, board members recognized that by thinking of this as an exception, they had created a new rule. "We learn from the past, but we can't change the past," a physical therapist on the board summarized, "We can say okay this time, but from now on we're going to do this."[26]

The IRB's struggle over this individual protocol had broader implications, in the minds of board members. "I'm surprised how long the conversation has lasted," a psychologist reflected, prompting weary chuckles from his colleagues. "But I think it was a good (conversation) because what comes of it is, I think, is a new policy. It's not going to apply just to [the investigator's] research, but to anybody else who does this kind of stuff, who wants to go back to participants. So I think it's really cool."[27]

The June meeting of Greenly State showed how this "new policy" entered board members' repertoire as an exemplary decision that could guide future studies. A new investigator in physical therapy planned to keep enrollment information on his subjects, and to Nathan this looked distressingly familiar. Nathan wondered whether the investigator kept the information because he intended to recontact these subjects, but the investigator assured the board that this information would be used solely to help compare data from other subjects to the data he hoped to collect in his proposed study. "That's fine," Nathan concluded. "I got a bit scared the last time we had a meeting about the other uses of information you keep during the course of a study," he explained. If the investigator wanted to contact participants in the future, he would have to tell them now.[28]

Creating local precedents was time-consuming for board members, and they often pursued issues for unpredictable reasons, such as a board member's personal conviction or a research subject's complaint. Once settled, however, IRB members used these decisions in a systematic way to guide future decisions. In this way, the boards that I observed standardized the types of problems they identified and the changes that they required to protocols, such as the units in which radiation levels should be expressed, how psychological inventories should be described to subjects, and the number of years for which a study's approval could be renewed, to name a few. The effects of these local precedents were twofold: first, established precedents allowed board members to make subsequent decisions more quickly without rehearsing settled debates, and, second, the precedents allowed members to defend their decisions on the grounds that they were imposing a consistent local policy.

Conclusion: Decision by Analogy

IRB members identify new problems somewhat idiosyncratically. For these problems, board members develop remedies to fit the particular instance and draw on the warrants of experts who happen to be at the table. But IRB members also use these decisions as prototypes that they apply to subsequent protocols, creating local precedents. When board members identify a problem in a new study proposal (or an element of it, such as the consent language or the research design), they do not try to apply general rules afresh to the specific case; rather, they apply the solution they came up with for a previous study to the new case at hand. Thus, local precedents are stock decisions, which board members use to manage subsequent protocols and speed future reviews. The decisions that establish local precedents are idiosyncratic, but once made, an IRB's decisions are quite stable and predictable over time.

This description of how IRBs make some decisions contrasts with the assumption that expert bodies deliberate within the framework of what has been called legal positivism. In this view board members are thought to apply fixed regulations to specific protocols with more or less accuracy, resulting in objectively right and wrong decisions. It is worth noting that many such analyses of IRBs are written by medical and health researchers, who in their main areas of research tend to aspire to the positivist ideals of experimental methods. However, their experimental style of reasoning, to use Ian Hacking's phrase, does not characterize how IRBs reach decisions.[29]

The way IRBs work, as I have described them, resonates more closely with what historian John Forrester, in his extension of Hacking, has called analogical reasoning. Forrester argues that "thinking in cases" stems from a pragmatic, not an experimental, tradition that was developed in Anglo-American law and medicine during the late nineteenth century. "If you think that invoking principles will avoid this method of reasoning," Forrester writes with particular reference to case-based decision making in modern medical ethics, "a skeptic of the relevance of your principles will soon require you to make explicit the exemplar, the prototype, the analogue onto which the invocation of your principles is grafted."[30]

Overturning the received wisdom about how IRBs make decisions helps explain several puzzles about these expert bodies, such as the way board members described their colleagues to me. IRB members valued experienced colleagues for providing the board's institutional memory, and they reported that new members (and they themselves) had to serve on the board for roughly a year before they were competent reviewers. I take these to be descriptions of how IRBs maintain continuity over time through case-based learning. As historian Thomas Kuhn has argued, people learn how to recognize and solve problems in a new field of study not by memorizing abstract rules. Instead, they are taught how to solve model problems—what he called exemplars—which allows them eventually to internalize the tacit knowledge and the thinking skills common among members of the field.[31] Through these model problems, students learn to distill an essential point from a mass of irrelevant details and figure out what constituted an appropriate question in the first place. Similarly, IRB members use exemplar protocols and problems as sources of model decisions that allow them to "do ethics"—to identify a subsequent protocol's essential problem amid all of its particulars, to recognize its similarity to a prior case, and to make a consistent decision. If IRB members were always applying general rules to particular cases, as some critics assume, rather than working from case to case, it is not clear what would be worth remembering or learning over time. Certainly, members pass on and become fluent with norms of group participation.[32] However, it seems that experienced board members also pass on the substance of prior decisions to new members, who have to learn at least some of the group's local precedents before they feel competent as reviewers.

Understanding group decision making in terms of case-based reasoning also helps explain why some IRBs belabor decisions that other boards make more quickly. Critics and regulators often attribute this variation in efficiency to an uneven distribution of material resources. I do not dispute that if a board has more full-time staff and funding, it will make speedier decisions. I want to add, however, that differences in boards' turnaround times are in part due to differences in their conceptual resources. As I have shown in the previous sections, settling contentious questions is time-consuming for IRBs: members distill a distinctive case to what they see as its central problem, then debate the proper decisions according to their individual sensibilities. It seems likely that differences in boards' decision-making efficiency with a given protocol depend on whether members have already established precedents to manage the concerns at hand. For example, the drawn-out deliberations of an IRB made up of medical researchers when faced with a qualitative study may not reflect hostility toward qualitative methods. Rather, it may point to a conceptual gap in the precedents readily available in board members' imaginations to deal with the type of concerns that they feel the study raises. Indeed, sociologist Carol Heimer links the speed of case-based decisions to the existence of precedents. She argues that thinking in cases requires a regular flow of instances that can be seen as examples of a prior case and that inefficiencies crop up in situations when "case streams do not exist . . . [such as] when something is being encountered for the first time."[33]

On a practical level, understanding how case-based reasoning affects IRB deliberations points to ways in which local boards might eventually coordinate their decisions across different institutions. A simple infusion of staff members and funding will not erase the variation across IRBs that trouble many investigators, especially those conducting multisite studies. Investing more time and money in human-subjects review will, rather, improve the speed with which IRBs continue to arrive at dissonant decisions. Consolidating boards will serve to decrease the number of idiosyncratic IRB decisions investigators have to manage but will not eliminate these particularities altogether. IRBs would make more similar judgments if local boards shared decision-making precedents at a national level. Given that IRBs make decisions based on cases, the challenge for a coordinated review system is not to craft more detailed federal regulations, but to train IRB members with a common set of real cases on which boards can base their decisions, as an alternative to local precedents.

It was a fortunate decision, but by no means a foregone conclusion, that the IRB at the University of Wisconsin, Madison, approved Devah Pager's protocol when it came to the board in 2001.[34] Pager was the researcher behind the employment and incarceration study in Milwaukee described at the beginning of this chapter. She had heard from other researchers that the Brandeis University IRB categorically refused to approve this kind of study design. It was felicitous that the University of Wisconsin IRB had no local precedent of its own, and so its members assessed the study with fresh eyes, which turned out to be sympathetic. They did require one change, though. Pager had planned to debrief employers after the study, in keeping with a more conservative reading of the regulations. The board members asked her *not* to debrief her research subjects. There was little risk of harm to participants, they reasoned. And if employers never knew they were in the study, then they would never be able to sue.

THREE

Documents and Deliberations: An Anticipatory Perspective

Anticipating Documents

In the end, the outcome of one IRB review turned on a remark about how the decision-making process would be documented. In this instance, Nancy, the Greenly IRB administrator, mentioned to a board member, "The minutes don't record you personally."[1] Why was this seemingly quotidian remark relevant to the board member? It reminded him that the meeting minutes erase members' personal accountability. For declarative bodies, documents are tools that members use to smooth interpersonal relationships and to invent a new social actor, such as "the IRB."

As a result, documents such as meeting minutes do more than chronicle decisions. By watching IRB members at work, I saw that the choices they made when evaluating studies were in part the product of how the process was recorded. To be sure, the decisions of declarative bodies—whether college admissions committees, funding panels, editorial boards, or IRBs—depend also on the quality of submissions, as well as on interpersonal power dynamics, differences in members' rhetorical skill, and happenstance.[2] However, the physical documents that board members eventually produce also play a central, if subtle, role in what will become their final decisions. As counterintuitive as it may seem, the end products of deliberations—namely, IRB documents—alter the decision-making process as it is under way.

To illustrate, I will compare two accounts of IRB meetings: one account that is given in the meeting minutes and another that is offered in my audio recordings of IRB deliberations. In this chapter, I follow the ethics review of two studies, one from Greenly and one from Sander State. In other words, I will look at decisions as they took place over time and as these events were formally documented afterward.

How to Do Things with Documents: Two Perspectives

Declarative bodies work toward consensus, as chapter 1 explains, because individual knowledge experts have no power on their own. Members of IRBs and other similar groups have legal authority (however tentative and contested) from the government only to the extent that they can act as a unit. There are barriers to collective agreement, however. Group members have competing interests, different standards of evaluation, and unfamiliar ways of justifying opinions. When individual group members differ in their views—or recoil at their colleagues' styles of presenting their views—it poses a problem for the group as a whole.

Enter the administrative document. Philosopher J. L. Austin, in his now-classic lectures "How to Do Things with Words," argued that people who are authorized to act on behalf of the state, for example by performing marriages, can invent new social realities with their spoken pronouncements. Austin, who was exploring language as an action, focused on the spoken word. He did not explore how this magical power might depend on material artifacts.[3] Words on paper, however, bolster the authority of spoken words. And, as I suggest in this chapter, people's knowledge that their words will appear on paper also changes what they are willing to say. Often recording people's views tempers extreme opinions, but in the case of closed settings such as IRB meetings, documents encouraged people to accentuate their more extreme views, because they could not be held personally accountable by those not present.

Administrative laws are the nuts-and-bolts rules that spell out how to govern. Among other things, administrative laws set requirements for how declarative bodies, such as IRBs, should record their decisions. For the government to achieve legal authority, as theorist Max Weber aptly described, "administrative acts, decisions, and rules are formulated and recorded in writing, even in cases where oral discussion is the rule or is even mandatory."[4] True to kind, in the case of IRBs, the Code of Federal Regulation instructs boards to produce meeting minutes that record "attendance at the meetings; actions taken by the IRB; the vote on these actions including the number of members voting for, against, and abstaining; the basis for requiring changes in or disapproving research; and a written summary of the discussion of controverted issues and their resolution."[5]

It goes without saying that meeting minutes give a simplified version of complicated events. Yet meeting minutes do not merely give abridgments; they give accounts of events that have been abridged in particular ways. I am interested in what is lost and what is gained in the space between talk and paper.[6]

Formal administrative documents (such as social surveys, patient histories, consent forms, and prison intake records) help to constitute new types of people (Americans, the diseased, subjects, and deviants).[7] This *constitutive perspective*, as I think of it, explains that administrative documents force people to identify as a given type—often as part of an effort by scientists and state administrators to compare and accumulate information about people and events across time and location as part of modern statecraft. As a result, documents subtly encourage us to adopt the terms provided by science and the state when we think about ourselves and others. That is to say, new social actors are brought into being through the identities, roles, and assessments provided to people through administrative documents. This chapter shows that documents—in particular, meeting minutes that are required by federal human-subjects regulations—invent "the IRB" as a unitary social actor.

When social actors are constituted in administrative documents, they are also placed in a story line. Documents give an official account of events that puts all relevant readers and relationships on the same page, both literally and figuratively. It is curious to observe that, in practice, administrative documents tend not to be particularly effective in fulfilling their purported aim of organizing and keeping track of people. Records and forms are often incomplete or haphazard, but these gaps should not be understood only as errors in documentation. Omissions and open-endedness in formal records reflect ongoing stories about people who are bound together by administrative documents (such as researchers and IRB members). In his influential study of patients' clinical records at the UCLA Medical Center, sociologist Harold Garfinkel described the documents there as bad enough to make one wonder "why 'poor records' as poor as these should nevertheless be so assiduously kept."[8] Garfinkel eventually argued that "bad" records were actually tools that helped their readers understand the past and the potential future of a clinician's relationship with a patient as, in his words, "a reconstructable record of transactions between patients and clinical personnel."[9] That is to say, formal documents always provide an idiosyncratic version of past events and of potential future actions despite the deceptively objective, authorless style of most official records.[10] Similarly, this chapter shows how IRB meeting minutes provide a selective reading of board deliberations that erases disagreements among IRB members, as well as board members' contestable reasons for making particular requests for changes to the research.

But meeting minutes do even more. I found that board members invoked the meeting minutes of their current deliberation—before the minutes had been written—in an effort to manage their relationships with each other and with researchers. This move is an example of a new *anticipatory perspective* for studying documents as social artifacts. IRB members used their knowledge of how their deliberations would be recorded to alter their deliberations as they were under way—and thus to shape the very decisions that the documents eventually record.

One consequence of using a document *in potentia* as a discursive tool is that it changes the course of IRB members' deliberation. In other words, by discussing the meeting minutes before the document has been created, board members pursued different courses of action and, consequently, reached different decisions than they would have if their deliberation had been documented in a different way.

Comparing Documents and Deliberations: Two Studies

The IRBs at Greenly and Sander had the typical structure, but both boards followed one uncommon practice compared to most IRBs: administrators invited the researchers under review to IRB meetings. In some instances, reviews were scheduled only if the researcher was going to attend the meeting.[11] To my mind, this makes their meetings all the more useful to study. If any ethics review could seem "transparent" and inclusive, it would be those carried out by boards that made a concerted effort to involve the researchers themselves.

The meetings of Sander State and Greenly IRBs had a routine: the researchers sat outside the meeting room until the administrators collected them at the preset time. The researchers then fielded questions from the IRB members. Afterward they left so that board members could further discuss the studies. The meaty issues were brought up and resolved in the boards' deliberation and final discussion stages, after the researchers had gone and before the vote. Although administrators did tally yeas and nays, voting was largely a symbolic exercise. In short, votes brought no surprises because the review ended when they had reached consensus. After the meeting, board administrators typed their handwritten notes into meeting minutes that were kept on file, and then they sent formal letters to the researchers based on the meeting minutes. The minutes and the letters described what, if anything, the researcher would need to change before the board would grant approval.

Greenly IRB: A Successful Attempt to Change a Study

I want to start by fleshing out a deliberation that I introduced in previous chapters. The review was of a planned study at Greenly University called

"Teaching Children to Manage Emotions." It seemed from the outset as if approval of the study would be "pretty straightforward," in the words of the board chair.[12] A professor of education who was near the end of a long, distinguished, and lucrative research career at the university was leading a study of preschool children at a local day care for low-income families. Her aim was to assess whether children would express their feelings in ways that teachers found more appropriate after the children had taken an expert-designed behavior-training course. The point of the course was to prepare children behaviorally for school, and the goal of the researcher was to promote the course nationwide if it proved effective. To control for any effects that the children's family background might have on their behavior, the parents who consented to the study would be observed with their children and these parents would be given several psychological tests via interviews. Their children would also be observed individually to allow researchers to gather various measures of development. After that, half of the children would take the six-month course during their time at the day care, and the other half would serve as the control group by continuing day care as usual. At the end of the course, the tests would be administered again to see if the children who had taken the course improved. Prior to the meeting, three IRB members had prereviewed the study: a professor of exercise physiology and a young clergyman had recommended approval without revision; a physician had asked the investigator to tone down the tantalizing language about parents' compensation and raised three points of clarification about how the study would be run. The primary investigator, named Dorothy, came to the IRB meeting at her appointed review time and brought along her junior faculty coinvestigator, who described the project at the beginning, fielded many questions about the study, and occasionally amplified board members' comments by repeating them into Dorothy's ear (she was hard of hearing). Compared with other reviews, the discussion with these researchers ran long, but when they left they seemed to have satisfied the physician's preview criticisms by agreeing to a few changes and to have placated other board members who had raised concerns during the discussion. The board chair told the researchers before they pushed back from the conference table, "I think you responded to all the questions that I know of."[13] This was the last face-to-face exchange between Dorothy and her colleague and the board members.

Despite the positive signs, however, the review of this project was not as straightforward as the board chair had anticipated. The board eventually approved a revised version of the study, but the go-ahead came several months after the researchers' visit. Board members discussed the study for the first time immediately following the researchers' visit, and after that discussion, the board asked for revisions. Board members then discussed the revised study at the next month's meeting and agreed to approve a future version of the study once the researchers submitted another round of revisions. The design of the study was not the enduring problem; rather, the way in which the researchers explained the study to parents.

The minutes of both of the meetings in which the study was discussed stated that the IRB's problem rested specifically with the "consent form" for parents. The meeting minutes also made plain that the researchers were being asked to revise several word choices in the consent form. I am going to focus on one requested revision in particular, which is the last bulleted point in the minutes from the day the study was first discussed (figure 1). This account of the deliberations explains that "the Board tabled any decision" until the researchers provided it with a revised consent form that included "a brief description, in lay language, of each of the measures" that researchers would be taking of parents and children.

How does this account of actors and events compare with the account offered in meeting transcripts? Immediately after the researchers left the first meeting, a thread of discussion began that stretched across several board meetings. You may remember from chapter 1 that Kevin, a psychologist on the IRB, outlined what he took to be a dire ethics problem that he had not directly raised with the researchers. According to him, what the researchers were pitching to board members and to parents as a measure of vocabulary was, in fact, an IQ test. When a straight-shooting kinesiologist on the board, Ted, paraphrased Kevin's point, "So, you're saying that she's misrepresenting what the tests are actually measuring?" Kevin replied that she was "not misrepresenting; just not stating."[14] Recent criticisms of IRBs tend to portray boards' requests to change words as petty caviling: requesting small word changes are ways that boards exercise symbolic power, the argument goes. This position overlooks, however, the fundamental changes in study procedures—and thus potential research findings—that word changes can make. The board members at Greenly, for example, discussed in the meeting that making Dorothy change the description of her vocabulary measure was not simply semantic but would have practical consequences such as decreasing study enrollment, delaying the start of research, creating additional work for the researchers, and provoking ill will toward the IRB. What could compel board members to force what they regarded as a consequential change to study procedure when many members aspired to focus on the ethics and leave the science to the investigator?

Review Board."

- Provide a check box for pare ts/guardians to in icate if they do not want to participate.
- Clarify the issue of confidentiality so that it is clear who will receive the data, how the data will be used, and for how long it will be kept.
- Provide information on the benefits of the study. This might include referral for further evaluation if testing shows any developmental delays.
- Delete the first sentence of paragraph 4, making the tone less absolute.
- Clarify the amount of time involved in the study.

4. ▉▉▉▉▉▉▉▉▉▉▉▉▉▉▉▉▉▉▉▉▉▉▉▉▉▉▉▉▉▉▉▉▉ presented a summary of the research. The Board tabled any decision on this protocol until the revised consent form is submitted. The revisions need to address the following issues.

- Clarify in the letter to the control group that "Although your child is not directly involved in the emotions course at ▉▉▉▉▉▉▉ we would like to ask your permission to...."
- Reference guardian as well as parent where applicable.
- Provide a check box for parents/guardians to indicate if they do not want to participate.
- Clarify that parents/guardians will receive $50.00 for each of the one hour sessions for a total of $150 every six months.
- Provide a statement that says "If in any of our evaluations or questionnaires, your child's responses are outside a normal range, we will notify you so that you may seek further evaluation."
- Revise the first paragraph on page 2 of the consent so that it is less absolute. This could be done by deleting the first two sentences and beginning the paragraph with the sentence "Parents and children enjoy working with us."
- Indicate how long the data will be kept.
- Provide an attachment which gives a brief description, in lay language, of each of the measures.

Figure 1. IRB meeting minutes from Greenly University.

The "modifications" that board members require to any given study are the products of their evaluations not only of the content of the study but also of each other's credibility in advocating certain types of changes.[15] During the deliberation on "Teaching Children to Manage Emotions," Kevin told board members about his own professional experience of developing the very instrument that researchers planned to use in the study. He suggested that he understood the nature and implications of the test better than anyone else on the board. Using the technical term for the measure of a person's so-called general intelligence, Kevin explained that what the researchers claimed was a vocabulary test for the parents was "the best G estimate of intelligence from one subtest from the [Standard Intelligence Scale]. And that's what she's giving. She's getting IQ on the parent."[16] Kevin explained that vocabulary qua IQ was "an important piece of information about an individual" and "almost as serious" as getting genetic information using "a blood stick that no one's told you about."[17] He encouraged board members to make the researchers give parents a fuller description of each of the psychological tests, which would include the contested vocabulary-IQ measure, and to provide parents with sample questions so that their consent could be better informed.[18]

My aim is not to rule on whether Kevin's understanding of the test is accurate or his description fair. Instead, I want to point out that Kevin's story about his professional experience was a language strategy that knowledge experts use to try to persuade listeners to agree with their points of view by describing why and demonstrating that they have authority in such matters. As I explain in chapter 1, Kevin's view was not the only viable position among board members. A more sympathetic view of the study came from Nancy (the IRB administrator), who often commented on education research that came to the board, based on her personal experience in sending her own children and grandchildren through various local programs. In this case, Nancy volunteered, "I understand [Dorothy's research program] is very good" in terms of the positive effects the courses had on children.[19] Nancy also suggested why Dorothy's research team might describe the tests to parents rather loosely, and explained, "I know from her previous experience with a lot of this, she doesn't want to frighten people."[20] As listeners, other IRB members played an essential role in authorizing or rejecting their colleagues' claims to have special insight into a study, judging whether an investigator must change research plans on the basis of that special insight.

In this case, most board members at Greenly (including Nancy, eventually) treated Kevin's claim to professional experience as most credible, and in so doing they solidified his views as the most authoritative in the evaluation of this study. For example, after Kevin reiterated his position that the researchers should describe the vocabulary measure to parents as an IQ test, Ted responded, "I think that's right. She has consent for vocabulary but not for IQ."[21] The board chair also told Kevin, "I can see your point. . . . I looked at these [test] names and I didn't think about that [IQ]."[22]

Yet even as Kevin advocated his view, spelled out recommendations, and warranted his credibility to speak on the matter, he often pulled back—not in his certitude that the investigators were collecting data on IQ, but in his willingness to demand changes to the study, or as he put it, his willingness "to throw a monkey wrench into this (study)." The board chair responded to his vacillation:

CHAIR: It sounds like at a minimum she needs to better explain what the testing is and potentially what it entails, whether that's IQ or depression and so forth, so that people at least understand. Now the question is whether they will know which test is which. They're not going to because, I mean, [IQ Test Name] doesn't mean anything to anybody, except you.

KEVIN: That's right.

CHAIR: I mean, I shouldn't say that. Maybe it means something to somebody else here.

GROUP: h

CHARLIE (PHYSICIAN): It means something to all of us, we just don't know what! h

GROUP: h

CHAIR: That's because our IQ isn't high enough to know this! h[23]

This exchange marks a tension caused by the fact that, in order to evaluate research, IRB members necessarily claim knowledge of some sort about an area in which the investigator also claims expertise. The result during this meeting at Greenly was that Kevin interspersed his critiques of the study with encouragement that it should nonetheless go on as planned. He was reluctant to force changes to the study because he felt certain that Dorothy, a senior researcher, would know that he, a junior faculty member, was responsible for demanding the labor-intensive changes that would affect study enrollment. "My gut impression is that we don't necessarily want to stop this," he explained: "Because I'm the one who gets identified on this and I'm dead meat on this campus, just to let you know. And I know there'd be repercussions because with her—her chair calls my chair, et cetera, et cetera, et cetera. It's because I'm the only one here who can identify this."[24]

In this situation, the meeting minutes served as a remarkably useful tool to manage the relationship between Kevin, his colleagues on the board, and the researchers. Kevin had successfully persuaded his fellow IRB members that the researchers were measuring IQ, that IQ was a sensitive piece of information, and that changes to the study were imperative. Yet he simultaneously insisted that the investigator should not be asked to change study procedures because it might jeopardize his professional standing outside of the IRB. Kevin was not appeased until Nancy reminded Kevin, "The minutes don't record you personally."[25] The meeting minutes, as board members discussed, could describe changes general enough to conceal Kevin's pointed concern but specific enough to ensure that the researchers would have to elaborate on the test as he recommended.

The meeting minutes for this review were entirely typical in form and therefore very useful for board members in managing accountability in the review. Board members used the minutes as a tool that would deflect accountability from Kevin for requiring changes to the study before it could begin. In material form, the meeting minutes gave the title of the study and named the two researchers, which focused responsibility for the study on them. On the flip side, however, the meeting minutes invoked "the Board" as the single social actor involved in the decision (specifically, in this case, "The Board tabled any decision on this protocol . . ."). According to the meeting minutes, "The Board" was the united, uniform agent that acted in reviews. In other instances, the minutes explained that the board "discussed," and at times the board "approved." To deal with this potentially awkward linguistic form, in which one organizational actor requested changes from two individual researchers, requests for study changes were written as commands in the meeting minutes: for example, "Provide an attachment which gives a brief description. . . ."

The transcript of the deliberation, by contrast, offers an account of the study review that could be thought of as an exchange between Kevin and Dorothy along with her coinvestigator, with an audience of university colleagues backing and rejecting competing claims to expertise. In the meeting minutes, however, Kevin's acute sense of personal responsibility during the deliberation was obscured, and the story line of what happened during the meeting most likely did not fit with researchers' experiences of the event because the key debate developed after they had left. Thus, when compared to the deliberation transcript, the meeting minutes provided a distinctive, unintuitive account of the social actors who were linked and the events that transpired during the study review.

Sander State IRB: A Failed Attempt to Change a Study

A proposed pilot study at Sander State, called "Home Environment and Life Outlook" provides a vivid example of how one board member's strongly felt but ultimately unpersuasive views were translated into and managed through the meeting minutes. In the study, the researchers, who were from the Department of Human Ecology, planned to compare whether features of assisted-living group homes affected residents' perceived quality of life. The researchers intended to interview residents, all of whom had mild dementia, and to observe their homes and how they used them—for example, to see whether they had plants to water, small pets to feed, or yards to walk in. The study was given conditional approval on the day it was reviewed, which meant that the researchers would get full approval by addressing the issues summarized in the minutes. They did not have to submit a revised study.

The section of the meeting minutes that I explore is a statement that asked the researchers, "Please note that IRB discussion indicated concern over co-morbidity factors influencing methodology." This statement is revealing in what it includes, namely the suggestion of board members' disagreement with one another through a description of "IRB discussion." This statement is also curious in what it excludes: most consequentially, a formal demand that researchers change their study design. Finally, it is worth noting that this statement accompanied one of the few votes of resistance from a board member (an abstention on principle) that I saw during my year of observing deliberations.

During the study review, board members asked the researchers to fix a number of inconsistencies between the project description and the consent form, requests that proceeded easily. Two board members lingered on the issue of precisely how researchers would establish that the people with dementia were cognizant enough to give informed consent to participate in the study. Then Henry, a middle-aged board member, started the line of inquiry that eventually prompted him to refuse to vote on this study. Henry pointed out that there are many different health problems that cause people to have dementia, and he asked the researchers, "Are you interested at all about causations? Do they have any relevance? Or would they have any relevance to your assessment of whether or not [residents] like this place versus this place?"[26] In an exchange that lasted two or three minutes, the junior member of the study team, who was leading the research in practice but not on paper, repeated that their focus was on residents' perceived quality of life, not on the underlying causes of dementia per se.

Eventually, the IRB chair looked to the other board members and asked, "Anything else?"[27] This was a strategy that the chair used both to exhaust all of the possible questions that board members might have while the researchers were present and, as in this instance, to truncate seemingly inappropriate discussion. In other words, the board chair's question did not follow from a resolved debate; rather, it imposed an end to the discussion of whether disease etiology mattered in this study.

Henry resisted this attempt to close discussion. "I just had a concern that the categories that you're drawing would make causation (important for understanding) cognitive impairment," he began again. "And it would appear to me, just on the surface, and obviously I'm not a learned individual in this area, so (I'm trying to sort this out). It seems to me, there may be some bias introduced if one person's impairment is due to A causation versus B causation. There may be some bias in there."[28]

Consider how Henry presented himself and his credibility in voicing this critique. Henry's official status on the board was as a community member, because he was not employed by the university. Yet he had graduate training in biochemistry and had worked as a bench scientist, so board members often relied on his judgment (along with that of physicians on the board) when they reviewed clinical trials. At this moment, though, Henry did not warrant his credibility, but instead deferred to the researchers' expertise by claiming that he was "not a learned individual in this area." With this further questioning, the junior researcher, rather than claiming as before that the cause of dementia was irrelevant to the study, instead explained that the medical records of participants were too difficult to access because of privacy regulations for health information.[29] The IRB chair then directly called on a different board member, effectively giving the floor to another person and topic. The researchers soon left.

The IRB chair at Sander State also used a technique that made it easy to follow the creation of a formal account of the meeting. After researchers left meetings, he read back to the board members his notes on what had been decided in the researchers' presence, which the administrator would type verbatim, to use as the meeting minutes and to use in an official letter to the researchers that told them what "action" the board members had taken. Often, the board members had a common sense of what changes they had requested, and a vote followed smoothly. In this case, the board chair read back his minutes-in-the-making, and two board members moved to approve the study with the listed changes. As they were about to vote, however, Henry intervened. Noting that his concerns had been left out of the list of modifications, Henry explained why it was essential that board members agree to include his recommended change: that the researchers collect data on the cause of dementia for participants.

This time, Henry made the same critique of the study, but he warranted his view differently: he justified his opinion with his professional experience. "It's my own personal belief that the criterion for this population that she's working with is critical," he started. "And etiology is associated with causation of dementia. To my mind, from my experience working in this area, it can have an effect on how you look at life." His fellow board members were not persuaded:

HENRY (EXTERNAL MEMBER, BIOCHEMIST): Multiple sclerosis patients who have dementia, (they can't go anywhere) and they know that it's progressive and that their brains are shrinking. Their ventricles are getting larger, the substance of the brain is wasting away. Versus a (diabetic) patient who has had diabetes and over the years is starting to get diabetic dementia. Those two people have different outlooks on life. Whether /

NIGEL (LINGUIST): She's not interested in the cause; she's interested in the result, it seems to me. They're interested in the result.

SAM (PHYSICIAN): I don't think it makes a difference to her study.

HENRY: I think it does, because she's looking at: How do environmental effects within this environment in which they are housed affect their outlook? How does that affect them? How does that make them feel? I think if you have a disease that changes your outlook on life, and how you feel day-to-day, your outlook on how that environment affects you, positively or negatively, is (a factor). . . . Your disease changes your perception of your environment. It does.[30]

Board members continued to emphasize the investigators' expertise in this study area over Henry's expertise. His claim to "experience working in this area" did not appear to be compelling to board members for an interview-based study in human ecology. One social scientist on the board rebuffed Henry for "commenting on methodology," although board members often required changes in study design on the logic that researchers are obligated, at a minimum, to produce useful data to justify involving people in research at all. In this case, however, in response to Henry's assertion that the researchers would not get "useful" data, another board member defended the researchers. This former dairy scientist defended the investigators' prerogative to define their standards of research according to their discipline, rather than by Henry's competing ideals: "Doesn't the usefulness of the data depend on the type of knowledge that you're talking about? You might interpret the results of this research as being 'Well, it's useless because I don't believe that they screened out this and this and this.' And so your interpretation as a result might be quite different from someone else's. But it strikes me that with the methodology that they're using, it really doesn't matter too much as far as they're concerned."[31]

At the same time, the Sander board members were quite conciliatory toward Henry. Review boards tend to be remarkably collegial groups because members are often selected (out of any number of experts in their fields) for their ability to be civil during an activity defined by disagreement.[32] One board member at Sander told Henry he could "understand your concern," but at the same time he reminded board members that getting health information was not "practical" in this study and that the project was only a pilot study. In a similar spirit of mollification, another board member suggested, "Our board report could also just have an addendum that says 'Discussion indicates that we are concerned about the multi-disease (problem), and we discussed those as being influential on your study.' We could just say we're concerned."[33] A third board member then asked that everyone vote and move on.

In the end, the meeting minutes reproduced these final conciliatory words: "Please note that IRB discussion indicated concern over co-morbidity factors influencing methodology." This phrasing reads as much as a note to Henry as a point of information for the researchers. Indeed, the researchers would not have to change anything about their study after reading this sentence. They were not its only readers, though. Henry and the other board members would also read and endorse the minutes at their subsequent meeting. Thus the minutes served to manage relationships among board members in this case. It is revealing, in addition, that in six months of meeting minutes that I collected, this was the only statement that portrayed the Sander State IRB as anything but a single, unified social actor. In other minutes, readers would find "The IRB expresses concern . . ."; "The IRB suggests . . ."; in the future, "The IRB would like to discuss . . . ," and even "The IRB commends [researchers] for a well-prepared set of responses and well-thought-out rationale."[34] The exception in the case of Henry's critique highlights the rule: when board members endorse an individual's viewpoint, their consensus is implicit in their self-description as the IRB.

Conclusion: Two Perspectives Revisited

As I described them, the opinions that were eventually adopted as those of the IRB were outcomes of a process of consensus-building (see chapter 1). Yet individual board members' efforts to find support for their positions were left out of the meeting minutes. That is to say, the stories of how board members reached their decisions were not recorded—such as the arc of Kevin's warrant based on his professional experience and Nancy's counterwarrant based on her personal experience as a mother, grandmother, and local day care user, which she invoked to encourage approval of what she (in contrast to Kevin) saw as a helpful study for disadvantaged children by a well-intended researcher. If members' justifications had been recorded, one practical implication might be that readers of the minutes could contest the legitimacy of these justifications and the required changes based upon them.

One aim of formal records, however, is to invent impersonal, rational stories of how events transpired and authoritative instructions for how events should play out in the future. The seeming objectivity of a claim can become "stronger" or "weaker"—that is, it can be contested and settled to a greater or lesser extent—depending on who makes the claim, how the claim is warranted, and whether it is documented in a way that enables the claim to stand outside of any one person or context.[35] I drew on what I called the constitutive perspective to show that meeting minutes were made to tell a particular story about the deliberations that did not merely abridge events but gave an account that was distinctive in systematic ways: with different actors and different actions than appeared during deliberations. Meeting minutes portrayed IRBs as unitary social actors who evaluate studies. That is to say, individual board members' successful attempts at consensus-building during board deliberations are presented in the meeting minutes as the actions and opinions of "the IRB." As the constitutive perspective on studying documents would suggest, the people who figure prominently in state administration—whether patients, deviants, or IRBs—are most firmly endowed with social reality when they become fixed in administrative documents. It is tempting, as a result, to think of the relationship between deliberations and documents as exclusively one-directional, with people's actions being followed by records that are followed by further actions and so on forward through time.

However, the process of translation between deliberation and document actually moved in both directions. Recall Kevin's predicament during the Greenly IRB meeting. Despite his initial reluctance to become professional "dead meat" at the hands of a powerful researcher, he became willing to allow a substantial change to her study precisely because, as the board administrator reminded him, the minutes would not record him personally. The minutes would erase Kevin's role in pressing for the changes, and this in turn fueled his critique of the protocol, which ultimately altered the way the researchers carried out the study.

Likewise, at Sander State board members used the future minutes of their current meeting overtly to manage relationships as the deliberation was still under way. In this case, Henry had failed to persuade other members that they should adopt his opinion despite his deep and enduring conviction that the researchers should be made to gather additional health data on study participants. To finally close deliberation in the face of Henry's persistent reopening of debate, a fellow board member suggested that a nonbinding comment (ostensibly written to the researchers) be included in the minutes. It is worth noting that this board member phrased her suggestion during the deliberation in the form of meeting minutes, a so-called hybrid utterance, which is a way of conversing with people using the language of bureaucratic documents.[36] Specifically, she suggested that board members could "just have an addendum that says 'Discussion indicates that we are concerned about the multi-disease (problem), and we discussed those as being influential on your study.'" Intentionally composed in such a way that researchers did not actually have to alter their study plan, the meeting minutes were used in the deliberation to make a show of collective dissatisfaction—purportedly for the researchers' edification, but practically to manage Henry and to manage board members' ongoing colleagueship with him.

Board members were not only aware that their decisions would subsequently be documented. They were also alert to how the constraints of meeting minutes could be useful during deliberations. Exploring what I have called an anticipatory perspective on studying documents, this chapter has shown that board members used their knowledge of how the minutes of their current discussion would be written as a social resource. They used the future documents in the present to manage relationships—between each other and between themselves and researchers (figure 2). As a result, IRB members tended to talk about the future record of the deliberation at particularly contentious moments, especially when they felt obliged to articulate a board member's extreme and deeply personal viewpoint in a seemingly impersonal way.

Thus, for declarative bodies like IRBs, the work of making a decision depends on two languages: that of deliberation and that of documentation. And the process of translation between deliberations and documents moves in both directions. Meeting minutes not only recorded decisions and reproduced categories, standards, and narratives of evaluation that had been used in deliberations; the not-yet-written minutes also steered the course of decision making as the process was still under way.

As a result, the review process, which is intended to make researchers accountable for their studies by producing managerial records of their planned activities and required behavior, also obscures the agency (and thus, the accountability) of the individual actors who make up the boards. By suggesting that members "make up" the IRB, I want to make explicit that individuals not only constitute the boards; they also do the inventive work of harnessing their opinions to the collective authority derived from the

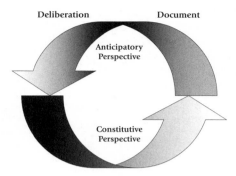

Figure 2. Two perspectives on documents and deliberations.

federal mandate of IRBs. Simultaneously and perhaps ironically, this process erased the accountability of individual board members.

For researchers who study living people, what is at stake in this process is nothing less than what can be known in the social sciences and biomedicine. When researchers look beyond the administrative burden of IRBs, they find that IRBs are important because they affect how researchers go about creating knowledge—and, as a result, the kinds of things that are knowable. IRBs rarely endorse or reject research proposals in their entirety on their first encounter with a potential study. Instead, IRB members suggest (read *require*) changes that a researcher could make to the proposal that would result in the board's approval. IRBs might suggest changes to researchers' site selection, sample size, recruiting methods, or interview questions, for example. But the administrative burden that researchers decry is not separate from the content and quality of IRB decisions. The documents enable board members' contentious decisions and sustain the impression that there is no *one* to hold accountable.

PART II

Setting IRBs in Motion in Cold War America

The IRB meetings that I observed were separated by many hundreds of miles, and yet the sites were uncannily similar: the oversized center table, the conference telephone as a focal point of the room, and the dependable reservoir of caffeine. But the setting is recognizable not only because of the features of the physical surroundings. The way IRB members made decisions was strikingly similar, as well. As part 1 of the book has shown, IRB meetings are recognizable because board members interact similarly, and they do so because boards are organized in the same essential way at different sites.

The National Institutes of Health started a human-subjects review board, the Clinical Research Committee (CRC), when its research hospital, the Clinical Center, opened in 1953. The CRC was the model for today's IRBs. The Clinical Center is the location of the story that unfolds in the next three chapters. It is the institution whose early review board structures the way that work gets done in IRBs today. To understand warrants, local precedents, and the ways the board members whom I observed anticipated and read IRB documents (chapters 1, 2, and 3), it is important also to understand why it ever made sense to have a group of experts judge a study rather than the researcher himself; why face-to-face conversations were valued more than written documentation, depending on the times and circumstances; and how this arrangement, which worked so tidily for enterprising researchers inside one federal building, spread to other sites across the United States and the globe.

The Clinical Center's review committee was not necessarily the first one. Researchers at other locations confronted the same problems that NIH researchers faced in the 1950s and 1960s, and so a few other universities and hospitals created similar committees around the same time. In this sense, the Clinical Center was not unusual. However, the creation of the CRC was unusually important because it was used as the model for today's IRBs. That is to say, it was the model that lawmakers picked up when Congress passed federal human-subjects regulations in 1974. As leaders of the nation's health research agency, the heads of NIH embedded within the regulations a model for making decisions—for governing with experts—that was familiar and that accommodated their existing practices.

Before reading on, it is worth getting a sense of the organizational structure to which the Clinical Center belonged. NIH is a U.S. federal agency within the Department of Health and Human Services (called the Department of Health, Education, and Welfare during the 1950s and 1960s). The U.S. Congress appropriates money to NIH each year, and NIH uses the money to fund health research. Importantly, NIH is not responsible for regulating research; it is responsible for conducting research.[1] There are two programs that NIH uses to funnel money to researchers. The first is the Extramural Program, which awards money from NIH to other institutions (universities, hospitals, and so on) after a researcher has submitted a successful grant application. When most people think of NIH research funding, they are thinking of projects sponsored through the Extramural Program, which are not physically located at the NIH campus in Bethesda, Maryland.

The second program through which NIH funds research is the Intramural Program. It has a small number of physical locations, the primary one being in Bethesda. If you drive down Rockville Pike outside of Washington, D.C., or hop off the Red Line at the "Medical Center" Metro stop, you will see the main campus of the Intramural Program.[2] This program pays the salaries of NIH employees, the building expenses of research facilities on the Bethesda campus, and all the other costs associated with running a research institution. Think of it as a university, except with less emphasis on courses and more on research. Whereas the Extramural Program is a pipeline for sending public research money to other sites, the Intramural Program is itself a set of research sites that center on one physical place, the main campus in Bethesda.

The Clinical Center is part of the NIH Intramural Program. If the Intramural Program is like a university, then the Clinical Center is like a university hospital. When you pass through security gates and go to the center of campus, you will find Building 10, also known as the Clinical Center. It was built relatively recently, in 1953, and so it was designed with the ideals of the modern hospital in mind.[3] The distinguishing feature of modern hospitals is that laboratories for research are down the hall from patients' rooms.

You can read contemporary theories of medicine and health care into the architecture of hospital buildings, and the Clinical Center is no different.

The phrase "bench-to-bedside" and the language of "translational research" capture what the Clinical Center architects were aiming for. Like the planners of other postwar research hospitals, the designers at NIH were trying to create a facility in which the things that chemists and molecular biologists were studying could be tried out in clinical research (in other words, research in hospital rooms on people). The new practice of placing patient wards and research laboratories next to each other served, in the words of Norman Topping, chairman of the Research Facilities Planning Committee, "to bring together in close physical and intellectual proximity the full array of high caliber laboratory and clinical investigators required for a broad attack on medical and related problems."[4] The hope was that advances in lab research would improve the everyday lives of Americans as quickly as possible through better patient care and preventive health programs.[5] That aspiration continues to inform federal funding priorities for health research today.

Trying out new research on people in hospital rooms was—and remains today—a thorny proposition. NIH leaders created a procedure for expert group review to enable and hasten research on human subjects at the Clinical Center in light of the political, ethical, scientific, and, it would seem, interpersonal problems that unfolded in the hospital during the 1950s. The men who served on the CRC brought the abstract procedure of ethics review to life. By the end of the decade, expert group review did not seem so novel, and Clinical Center researchers started attributing to expert group review a broader range of virtues. Researchers came to imagine it as a procedure with enough rhetorical and moral force that it could stave off lawsuits by human subjects. They were right. But as it turned out, lawsuits started coming at NIH from a different direction: as a result of studies funded through the Extramural Program. In the mid-1960s, NIH leaders decided that all universities, hospitals, and other research institutions needed CRCs of their own. It was a way to protect NIH itself from liability by placing legal responsibility for researchers on the institutions it funded through the Extramural Program.

Dr. James Shannon coordinated the creation of the CRC when the Clinical Center opened, and he was the man behind the 1966 federal policy that spread review boards across the United States. Shannon was, by all accounts, "a superb science administrator," and "a great 'bureaucrat.'"[6] Shannon's greatness as a bureaucrat—a superlative and a vocation that seem, by definition, to be incompatible—rested on his talent for delivering with equal conviction his personal beliefs and the strategic rhetoric suggested by advisers whom he directed behind the scenes. Shannon's tenure as NIH director coincided perfectly with NIH's good financial fortune: the NIH budget increased more than threefold in his first three years as director and did not diminish substantially until 1968, the year he left the directorship. Many scholars and former colleagues therefore link the "golden age" of NIH to Shannon personally.[7]

True to form, Shannon gave the National Advisory Health Council a proposal for the nationwide creation of IRBs in 1965, and the council obediently endorsed it. The next step fell into place, too. The job of the National Advisory Health Council was to advise the U.S. surgeon general, and so, on the council's advice, Surgeon General William Stewart announced in February of 1966 that all research institutions would have to set up a group-review procedure if they wanted to continue getting federal money. Nearly all universities, hospitals, and research agencies used at least some public funding to operate, and so essentially all set up local IRBs.

It is worth considering what the surgeon general told research institutions about the new requirement for expert-group review. They might have been relieved to learn, from a memo Stewart sent them: "The wisdom and sound professional judgment of you and your staff will determine what constitutes the rights and welfare of human subjects in research, what constitutes informed consent, and what constitutes the risks and potential medical benefits of a particular investigation."[8]

This memo established the institutional review system, a system built on expert discretion and local variability. The policy got teeth in 1974 when the group-review requirement graduated from policy to federal regulation. At that point, the rules were elaborated and became more enforceable, and in later decades the particular rules continued to be tweaked ("harmonized" and specified).[9] But February 1966 marks the moment when hospitals and universities picked up the model that had been crafted to accommodate the professional discretion valued by NIH researchers.

Thus the Clinical Center policy was lifted from that specific site and applied to virtually all universities and hospitals.[10] The Clinical Center was a peculiar place, though: physically, organizationally, and socially. To understand how IRBs work today, we have to come to terms with what makes them a distinctive way of making choices, which becomes apparent through a look back at the unusual site for which the policy was invented.

The chapters that follow cover two decades, from the late 1940s to the late 1960s, the period when the federal government reorganized its relation to science in America and became the greatest patron of research. There were strings attached to the federal money, however. Those strings were able to animate researchers in new ways—by inclining them toward particular topics of study and by guiding their everyday habits of work. One of the means by which the federal government influenced the way researchers worked was through research review.

FOUR

An Ethics of Place

The standards for medical practice established at the Clinical Center will be our own and not those of any other institution.

—Meeting minutes, Clinical Center Medical Board, June 9, 1953

Procedures and Principles

Carl Zimmerman was admitted to the Clinical Center in December 1954 and discharged more than two years later. By all accounts, he was a difficult patient. Carl defied doctors' orders, was "uncooperative and belligerent" with nurses, and managed more than once to get bitten by lab rats. Any sour feelings were mutual. Carl loathed the constant surveillance of his hospital room, the monotony of clinic life, and nurses' patronizing tones. During his years at the Clinical Center, he refined the art of retaliation, custom-made for a hospital setting. At the height of inspiration, Carl refused to get out of bed to get weighed, declined to collect his own stool samples, rejected meals, and hid himself in the bathroom. His subversive laziness proved quite effective in sabotaging doctors' plans. Carl seemed to sense that his body was his most valued resource at the Clinical Center, and so he used it as his truest weapon.[1]

Carl was deceitful, unreliable—and also perfectly healthy. As one clinician aptly put it: "Patient has no pertinent complaints," the operative word being "pertinent."[2] Carl was not malingering. Rather, he lived the better part of his early twenties at the Clinical Center as part of the Normal Volunteer Patient Program (often referred to as the Normals program). Through this arrangement, NIH admitted healthy people to the hospital alongside sick people. They were there to be studied.

By creating the Normals program, NIH redefined what it meant to be a patient. Inside the Clinical Center, a "patient" was not necessarily a person with an illness, as colloquial usage would suggest. Instead, a patient was a human site of medical intervention. Among the first patients allotted beds in the new hospital were men and women who, like Carl, were admitted *because* they were in good health.

Today, healthy people are admitted to hospitals every day as research subjects. The pay is good for higher-risk studies that require a stay in a clinic, so volunteers often think of it as a form of contract employment. These days, NIH still admits to the Clinical Center healthy people who would have been called Normals ("normal patients," "normal volunteers," or "normal controls") in Carl's day. These inpatients (and many more outpatients, who do not stay overnight) are now admitted through the program as "healthy volunteers," since the Normals program was tastefully renamed the Clinical Research Volunteer Program in 1995.[3]

Before the Clinical Center opened, doctors did not routinely hospitalize healthy American civilians.[4] Our present-day arrangement is remarkably different from a not-so-distant past when it was unthinkable to admit healthy people to hospitals—in part because it was unnecessary, but also because it would have been thought morally suspect. Since World War II, however, the reasons for hospitalizing people have multiplied through a series of small steps and everyday decisions by doctors, lawyers, and administrators. The hospital—a place where, until the nineteenth century, the sick went to die—eventually became a place where the sick might also be healed and, since the 1950s, a place where both sick and healthy civilians go to be studied.[5] This final shift took some doing, and, as doctors learned, it limited their ability to claim convincingly that the sacred doctor-patient relationship ensured caring treatment of their charges.

The ideal of the doctor-patient relationship did not fit well with the new kind of patients—namely, healthy patients—that researchers wanted to study at the Clinical Center when it opened in 1953. A new model of governing research at the Clinical Center, called "group consideration," helped make it possible for NIH to hospitalize and carry out research on otherwise healthy citizens. NIH leaders layered the practice of group consideration on top of the traditional model of doctor-patient decision making, which was first imagined for sick people and built into professional codes of ethics. The group-consideration technique gave decision-making authority to groups of doctors rather than to individual doctors alone.

NIH's guidelines for group consideration described a procedure, not a set of ethics principles. NIH clinical directors would meet in the Clinical

Center conference room and review studies that their colleagues planned. The practice improvised on existing work habits and built on familiar hospital routines. Inside the Clinical Center, group consideration fit with physician-researchers' experiences in other roles: as doctors on ward rounds, as grant reviewers in study sections, as members of animal-protection committees, and as warm bodies in myriad other committee meetings. Group consideration was not invented de novo, and yet clinicians used the old practices in a new way, to deal with a question previously left to individual doctors: how to be good to their patients.

The practice of group consideration was invented to manage practical problems and legal demands specific to the federal research hospital, to govern—and thus enable—research on healthy patients within the physical confines of the Clinical Center. To researchers, group consideration was an invaluable resource, because it freed them to admit nonsick people to the hospital. With some reluctance, NIH lawyers and department heads endorsed the group-consideration guidelines as official policy in 1953, an act suggesting to researchers that their plan had some legal traction. The policy was to apply narrowly to the goings-on inside the walls of the Clinical Center, given lawyers' fear of liability. Group consideration had a physical boundary, in other words, not an organizational boundary. If a researcher had a delicate instrument in another building on campus, it often had to be moved into the Clinical Center; the patient could not be moved to it. When a scientist proposed a research procedure at odds with group-review requirements, his colleagues pondered, in all seriousness, whether the Clinical Center boundary could be redrawn so that, technically, an inside wall would mark the policy's limit, rather than the building's external wall.[6]

Absorbed in the minutia of practical problems that group consideration helped to solve, NIH researchers hardly realized what they had done. The fathers of the Clinical Center had created an ethics of place. This was a new way of conceptualizing what an ethics policy was bound to. For centuries, professional organizations had created codes of ethics that attached to practitioners, that is, to individual people. The group-consideration policy, by contrast, was stamped on a building. NIH leaders intended this practice, like other local policies at the Clinical Center, to be their "own and not those of any other institution," as they reassured themselves in the politically treacherous days before the hospital opened in 1953.[7] Although they did not intend it at the time, group consideration became the model for the practice now known as institutional review. And NIH leaders enacted it with healthy human subjects in mind.

The Healthy-Patient Paradox

Healthy people have been indispensible to medical researchers for centuries. Prison inmates, for example, have been such a valuable resource for generations of researchers in the United States that Americans worked hard to defend this tradition—and were successful—even after the revelations of Nazi prison experiments and have continued to defend prisoner research today.[8] At NIH itself, researchers drove to nearby Jessup Prison in Maryland and Lorton Prison in northern Virginia to study inmates there, until a lawsuit and congressional hearings in 1973 persuaded them to stop.[9] (NIH also brought prisoners to the Clinical Center, as I explain in chapter 6.) In prison studies, researchers were often testing new drugs or vaccines. Starting in the 1930s, pharmaceutical companies kept new, untested therapies in ready supply for doctors, but the new remedies brought mixed results for patients. Penicillin and malaria vaccines were a triumph of World War II, thanks to government sponsorship of research and testing on healthy prisoners and soldiers. But toxic drugs and contaminated vaccines also killed unknown numbers of people during this period, and in 1962 Congress forced the Food and Drug Administration to tighten its regulations. For the first time, the FDA was required to track drugs, tighten testing requirements, and follow approved drugs on the market—or at least, that was the aspiration.[10]

In addition to changes in the field of chemistry, midcentury developments in physics altered American medicine. Starting in 1946, engineers in Oak Ridge, Tennessee, started mass-producing and shipping radioisotopes to researchers throughout the United States for use in medical research. After World War II, interested parties—from potentially unemployed nuclear engineers to members of the Harry Truman administration—glowed with the possibility that medical research might offer some positive peacetime use for one of the biggest by-products of the war: American nuclear infrastructure and know-how.[11] For their part, NIH administrators contrived to host human radiation research on behalf of the Department of Defense because, they argued, it would draw less attention than other sites.[12] For NIH, the claim to be important to national defense may have been a stretch, but it was a useful claim as the Korean War started to heat up. NIH guessed correctly that President Dwight Eisenhower and the Congress would direct funding toward anything done in the name of national defense. So it was that, during the early 1950s, NIH employees and healthy patients could be seen streaming out of the Clinical Center as they took part in drills to practice converting the hospital into a triage facility in the event that Communists dropped a nuclear bomb on Washington.[13] In another effort to

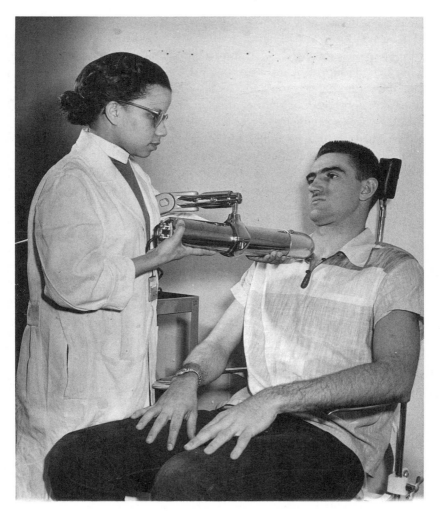

Figure 3. Thyroid study on a Mennonite Normal patient at the Clinical
Center, 1958. Courtesy of the Mennonite Church USA.

secure public funding for the new facility, NIH leaders also promised that the
Clinical Center would tackle the diseases of interest to Congress in the postwar years: cancer, heart disease, and mental illness. Layered underneath, in
addition, was an abiding concern with infectious diseases, given NIH's roots
in the Public Health Service. What these diseases had in common was the
tantalizing prospect of control through new drugs and nuclear medicine.

These shifts in chemistry and physics offered new tools for medical researchers and, as a consequence, prompted health activists and scientists to adopt new standards in what counted as a good, convincing answer to a research question. The most persuasive answers, scientists agreed, would take the form either of comparisons between sick and healthy people or of baseline observations of how drugs, nutrients, and hormones affected unsullied, well-working bodies.[14] Like their contemporaries, researchers at NIH latched on to these topics and these standards of evidence. Case in point: on his first day at the Clinical Center, Carl was enrolled in a toxicity study for the drug Natrinil, a potential therapy for congestive heart failure. On his last day, he was injected with a compound that had been tagged with radioactive carbon in a study of cholesterol.

What these new research standards in turn demanded, scientists felt, was that researchers bring healthy bodies into clinics, rather than taking mobile clinics to the healthy bodies. The imperative to host healthy people in hospitals was a distinctive feature of postwar medical research. Although researchers continued to try to recreate laboratory conditions inside prisons and schools and in military theaters, those were often far from ideal arrangements.[15] By 1950 the necessities of research simply did not travel well in many cases. Much of the equipment used for drug and radioisotope tracer studies was too cumbersome or delicate to move. Other research essentials, including radioisotopes and, later, psychotropic drugs, were illegal to transport without prior approval from other agencies.[16] As a matter of convenience and rigor, scientists preferred to have laboratories near patients. And, as NIH bookkeepers were ever aware, it was often cheaper to bring the healthy people to the research equipment. This explains why the Clinical Center was built with one square foot allotted to patients' rooms for every two feet of laboratory space.[17]

Yet the features of institutional life in which prisoners, soldiers, and wards of the state lived were part of their value. Researchers demanded a good deal of long-term, physical control over healthy subjects for drug screening, controlled trials, and baseline studies. The level of social engineering that was possible within these institutions was, in part, what made their residents coveted research material. Every aspect of their carnal experiences could be controlled: food, exercise, sleep, and sex. All of that, and the "clinical materials" (as the people were called) were low-cost and in large supply.

As a result, these useful features were built into postwar clinical research centers, to create the best of both worlds. Physically, places like the Clinical Center were built so that healthy subjects were down the hall from basic science labs. In their social design, research hospitals were organized so that patients could be tightly controlled and closely observed over long spans of time. When Carl was in a crucial phase of a study, for example, staff learned to suspend his pass privileges and watch him incessantly—not for drug reactions but simply to know his whereabouts at all times. Here he was playing cards with his roommate, and there he was entranced by the television in the library.

The aspiration of full control was never achieved. Carl was still able to slip out for late-night smokes and to eat illicit meals on other wards. And such close monitoring encouraged the very disobedience and secretiveness that it was designed to prevent. The night nurse on Carl's ward recorded in his chart that on January 18 at 2:00 a.m., after she had earlier reminded him to stop playing cards and go to bed, Carl "exploded" at her: "If you don't stop peeping in, you'll get something to be sorry for." The tight surveillance can be felt not only in the tone of this exchange but also in the simple fact that Nurse Fanning documented it. Battles over following rules veiled disagreements over who was in charge of patients—nurses, doctors, or patients themselves. On Halloween, for example, nurses denied Carl a pass to leave the Clinical Center because he had not requested it before 9:00 a.m., per hospital policy. Not to be outdone, Carl asked Dr. Haney, who gamely granted a pass. It would not affect the study at this point, Haney might have thought, if Carl had a few hours' relief from the brick and tile of the hospital, not to mention a distraction from the one-thousand-calorie diet of toast and jelly he was on. What did affect the study was Carl's phone call, five days later, explaining that he was outside of Gettysburg with a broken-down car. When Carl eventually turned up at the end of November, Dr. Haney scolded him, sent him to the Normals coordinator to discuss his shenanigans, disallowed him from leaving the nursing unit, much less the hospital, and promptly put him back on a one-thousand-calorie diet for his Nevilar study.[18]

Clinical Center leaders imagined that healthy humans would be the limiting resource for the type of research they considered a priority. The people who came to the new Clinical Center most eager to be admitted were inevitably turned away. Receptionists could count on seeing a small, steady stream of locals with rather mundane illnesses come into the front lobby: children with mumps, elderly people with bad hearts. The women at the front desk were trained to show concern, to explain that "only patients with the particular type of disease under study at the Center can be accepted," and to direct them down Old Georgetown Road to Suburban Hospital, where they could be treated.[19] Many Bethesda residents were vexed to learn that they could not use the new hospital that had strained schools, roads, and housing markets. "We are not concerned with filling beds just to have bodies in them," Dr. Joseph Smadel fumed during a low-occupancy crisis in 1958. "These beds are here for their use in research; clinical investigation."[20] From the time the Clinical Center opened, people with interesting diseases and people with no disease at all were the most coveted and were also in shortest supply.

Sick patients were transferred from other hospitals, but as a 1954 survey found, their "ideas of what the Clinical Center would be like prior to their coming here were predominantly negative. They frequently expressed fear of a 'cold, scientific place where the patients would receive little attention.'" Sick patients often acquiesced to the move because of "their confidence in their referring physician and their families' encouragement," the survey found. Patients were not necessarily drawn by the free care that NIH offered. To the contrary, the NIH associate director had urged the agency to bill patients in an effort to *encourage* them to come. A plan for national health care had recently failed under the Truman administration, tarred by enduring fear of socialized medicine. Indeed, the survey found that "if this was their first experience with free medical care, they were concerned about a 'catch in it' or having to pay later."[21] Bear in mind that in 1954, the year Carl arrived at the Clinical Center, Linus Pauling won the Nobel Prize in Chemistry and yet was denied NIH research funding because he, along with thirty other applicants, fell short on national "loyalty criteria" that were used in awarding grants.[22] It was with good reason that Clinical Center leaders fretted about recruiting enough patients. Just as revealing as the survey results themselves is the fact that NIH leaders were worried enough to take a survey.

NIH leaders saw the media as a powerful but potentially fickle ally in their recruitment efforts. Clinicians circulated positive press about studies in their effort "to get more of the kind of referrals of the type [of] patients" that they needed.[23] Information officers were put on the case, too. NIH invited media attention as long as its leaders could control the message—a difficult prospect.

Adding to NIH recruitment woes, Public Health Service regulations allowed little room to give interesting patients—sick or healthy—incentives to come to the Clinical Center. Patients would be considered objects of study first and last. "Work based only on the fact that the patient needs it for the improvement of his health would not be authorized," Edward Rourke advised the director of the not-yet-opened Clinical Center in 1951.[24] Rourke was a lawyer at the Public Health Service's Office of General Counsel who had been assigned responsibility for the Clinical Center as it began to take shape in 1950. Among other things, Rourke's job was to suggest regulations that would be good for the Clinical Center within the limits of the law—and within his own limits to defend scientists in the years to come. For his own sake, if not the sake of patients and doctors, Rourke wanted clarity in a few specific areas, and he took it upon himself to remove ambiguities. Rourke was worried about liability, naturally, and it was still unclear to him who would get sued if something went wrong in four situations: first, when patients were being moved to Bethesda from their doctor's care; second, when NIH clinicians moonlighted in a private practice; third, when clinicians treated patients at the Clinical Center for ailments that were not actually under study; and, finally, the persistent puzzler, when clinicians were doing things to patients for research alone, not for the improvement of their health.[25] Rourke's job was to flesh out rules and to explain to NIH scientists and administrators how they might translate federal law into everyday practices inside the hospital.[26]

In effect, Rourke was the law incarnate. And as Rourke understood the law, medical care at the Clinical Center could serve only a research goal. Anything approximating treatment was allowed only if the condition was "itself complicating and impairing the individual's value to [the] study." If a bed-ridden heart patient had trouble seeing, Rourke instructed, doctors could give him spectacles only if "assisting his vision may reasonably be said to contribute to his tolerance of his restrictions, and would thus better assure his cooperation in the study." If patients were too sick to be studied, clinicians should not treat them, but discharge them.[27]

Regulations also restricted, according to Rourke, "educational and recreational activity for non-therapeutic purposes," otherwise known as pleasure and edification. Still, Normal patients, at least, found ways to enjoy both. They played sports, fell in love, took classes, and worshipped on Sundays.[28] There were clubs and outings, in addition to vocational assignments, which enabled NIH to use Normals as labor and as objects of study during their stays. Many of Carl's contemporaries made an enviable life for themselves, including Bert, whom a counselor fondly described: "He reads a great deal, plays in [the] gym, golfs, goes to Gaithersburg to participate in church activities. [He] uses hospital activities a great deal for his own pleasure. We see him daily for one reason or another. He has no problem of getting away from everyone when he wants to. He works on the newspaper, parties, dramatic groups, etc. [He] dates Dana on 3W. There is much rivalry between the 3W girls for [his] attention."[29]

Still, living the good life at the Clinical Center was rare and so quite valuable to NIH administrators. Bert had "never had a problem of adjustment to the hospital or of what to do with his time," according to Ms. Donniger in the Social Services Department. "He is frequently used and interviewed when a control is needed to contact the outside community because he is well poised and good looking." Less than two months after Bert arrived, NIH administrator Irving Ladimer took him on a drive to a Normals recruiting event. Ladimer had a law degree, like Edward Rourke, but the men worked in different offices and, it is fair to say, were employed to use their law degrees to contradictory ends. Rourke and his colleagues in the Office of General Counsel were positioned to keep researchers reined in. Ladimer, by contrast, worked in the NIH research planning unit to spur research on. Throughout his career, Ladimer aimed to minimize restrictions on medical researchers, as later chapters explain. In the spring of 1954, Ladimer was in a car with Bert, who was taken to a recruiting event to vouch for the NIH Normals program because several volunteers had recently reneged on their promises to move to the Clinical Center. Dutifully, Bert testified alongside Ladimer that there was no coercion to be studied and that he had a lot of freedom to move around while living at the hospital.[30]

Even NIH planners anticipated that Normal patients would struggle to relocate and to live inside the hospital. As a result, the Clinical Center included a Social Services Department, whose staff regularly met with Normals and encouraged their theater troupes, glee clubs, work placements, and other activities to temper the sense of boredom, isolation, and confinement that the staff expected Normals to feel. During Carl's first months on ward 9-West, for example, he wept often. Soon after he arrived, Carl had started on a long-term, reduced-calorie rice diet led by Dr. Sandstead. Aware of Carl's sadness, Sandstead nonetheless "felt that patient was getting along all right and believed his problem to be loneliness and difficulty in finding companionship." Sandstead enrolled Ms. Byrd, Carl's social worker, as a surrogate friend. She arranged for Carl to repair equipment around the hospital, but he had "great difficulty controlling tears and seemed disturbed. He told [the supervisor] he had discontinued school and [had] failed at everything. He seemed unable to talk with her further."[31]

Carl's failures weighed on him intensely at this time because he thought, after only a few months at the Clinical Center, he was on the brink of failing again: he wanted to be released from the rice-diet study. Clinicians were expected to do a certain amount of "wet-nursing" with Normals during their first experiences in a big town—not to mention their first time living in a hospital.[32] Whatever the reason, Carl's personal anguish caused a crisis for Sandstead, as well, who "wondered how long [Carl] might be able to continue and whether the research plans might be jeopardized. Dr. Sandstead recognized patient's disturbed state and requested worker continue in sup-portive role." Conveniently, a NIH psychiatrist determined that it would be in Carl's best interest to stay on the study because "such a rigid diet with the attending personal restrictions met some of patient's needs to suffer, to pay for what he gets and the prestige in that he felt the rice diet was the most difficult that anyone could be on. He commented a number of times that he would never go on the rice diet again, although Dr. Sandstead wanted him to go on it for a longer period after he had a chance to rest." It is not clear that it helped the veracity of the data: Carl defied the laws of physiology by gaining weight on the diet, and the mystery of his persistent stomachaches was solved when he confessed to bingeing on a bag of candy. But Sandstead did persuade Carl to stay on the study by appealing to the greater good of science, the betterment of "the Asiatic people," the strength of his own char-acter, and—the clincher—the concession that Carl could take a vacation at the end. Often the greatest reward for staying in the Clinical Center was finally getting to leave.

The Guinea Pig Units

From the vantage point of 1951, Clinical Center leaders worried about what would draw patients to the hospital. Sick patients, they reckoned, could be transferred from other clinics (although local doctors resented the presump-tion that they would send their most interesting patients to the Clinical Center so that NIH researchers could study the diseases). Clinical Center planners feared that healthy patients would be harder to come by, given that, legally, there were few incentives to offer patients. The long tradition of self-experimentation and of experimenting on medical trainees continued. But researchers wanted a bigger pool, and there was a new ban on using NIH employees as human subjects. (The administration worried that service employees would volunteer in studies to avoid work.)[33] To deal with the problem, NIH leaders turned to the Selective Service.

In 1951 clinical leaders began piecing together what became the Normal Volunteer Patient Program, out of the remains of a World War II program that created "Guinea Pig Units." At the time, the Clinical Center was just an elaborate mirage hovering over the field where NIH softball teams squared off, and World War II had barely faded from memory. During the war, Carl's church and other "historic peace churches" had created the National Service Board for Religious Objectors to place parishioners who had been drafted in noncombat military service.[34] Coincidentally, medical research-ers working in behalf of the war effort needed large primates, including humans, for medical studies that would ultimately protect soldiers. Until the early 1940s, military research on dogs, horses, and monkeys was heavily restricted in response to the antivivisection movement.[35] And animal models did not always translate smoothly onto humans. These two factors made soldiers seem to be a good alternative. Some worried, however, that research on healthy soldiers was a poor use of resources and was possibly counterproductive if the research compromised their performance on the battlefield. Sick servicemen were another option. During World War II, marines were studied as they convalesced, a policy that changed in 1944 when the military restricted doctors from studying war casualties in government sickbeds.[36] One heart researcher, Dr. Luther Terry, faced restrictions on studying men who were admitted to the Baltimore Marine Hospital. With the Clinical Center set to open, Terry moved to NIH, where he became the first chairman of the Clinical Center's Medical Board and admitted Carl to the facility in 1954. In Bethesda, Terry enjoyed his new access to hospitalized human subjects for his research on hypertension.[37]

The Medical Board of the Clinical Center was a group of roughly a dozen men who created policy for the Clinical Center. The Clinical Center director established the board in 1952 and hosted meetings down the hall from the NIH directors' office before the building opened. The board was made up of the top researchers of all the institutes, often the clinical chiefs and institute directors. They were a close-knit group of researchers and administrators, and they got together every other week in their role as members of the Medical Board.

In short, the elite, old-guard researchers were also the Clinical Center policymakers. For example, Dr. Luther Terry was rewarded for his successes as a researcher with higher positions of administrative authority at NIH. He moved up the ranks of the National Heart Institute through the 1950s and was eventually President John Kennedy's pick for surgeon general in 1961. Terry's crowning achievement came in 1964, when, despite his southern heritage, he announced as surgeon general that smoking caused cancer.[38] Throughout his government career, Terry remained committed to the ideal of scientific freedom. And as chairman of the Clinical Center's Medical Board in 1953, he was in the right place for such a commitment.

The Guinea Pig Units—the churches' term, not the military's—were relatively small and were established relatively late in the war. Launched in 1943, the program funneled more than one hundred religious objectors into labs and hospitals across the United States before the war ended. A few men were placed at Goldwater Hospital, a facility marooned on New

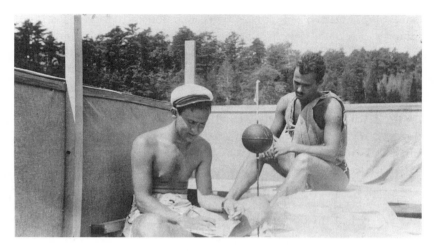

Figure 4. Two members of the Friends church, who were conscientious objectors during World War II, served in a study of sea saltwater effects at camp 115.10, Massachusetts General Hospital. Courtesy of the American Friends Service Committee and the Center on Conscience and War, Peace Collection, Swarthmore College.

York City's Welfare Island (sensibly renamed Roosevelt Island in 1972). From this site, doctors studied, for example, how long soldiers could be expected to survive after a shipwreck with varying amounts of food, water, and warmth.[39]

Inside the hospital wards, men were also infected with malaria so that researchers could compare new drugs developed to treat the disease.[40] Malaria was debilitating Allied troops (as well as residents of the American South), and antimalarial drugs became a major topic of study after the Japanese blocked the supply of Americans' main therapy, quinine.

Dr. James Shannon was the link between World War II's Guinea Pig Units and their postwar incarnation at the Clinical Center. During the war, Shannon had played two roles—one as an influential university scientist and the other as a powerful government administrator—both of which made him aware of researchers' indebtedness to conscientious objectors as "clinical material."[41] As associate professor of medicine at New York University in Manhattan, Shannon directed the school's clinical research service, which consisted of one hundred beds at Goldwater Hospital, an "extraordinary resource" for medical researchers at the time.[42] There, Shannon and his staff developed and compared new malaria drugs (as well as therapies from other labs), using the conscientious objectors living at Goldwater in his

Guinea Pig Unit. In his funding requests, Shannon asked for (and received) money to pay the wages of his technicians, research assistants, and nurses, as well as the conscientious objectors.[43]

On the national level, Shannon oversaw a network of researchers who were testing new malaria drugs on healthy men. The U.S. Office of Scientific Research and Development ran wartime research efforts, which included the Board for the Coordination of Malarial Studies to tackle the new disease threat. During the war, Shannon served as chair of the board's Panel on Clinical Testing. In his lab notebooks, he recorded data on hundreds of men who had been infected with malaria, noted how acutely ill they became, grouped them according to the drug administered to them, and tabulated the days that elapsed before they recovered—not only at Goldwater, but at sites across the United States under his purview.[44]

When Shannon accepted a top job at the National Heart Institute in 1949, he transplanted not only the group of young researchers he had cultivated at Goldwater, but also the idea of the Guinea Pig Units. By this time, Shannon was a well-respected administrator and scientist—in that order. (During the war, Shannon had actually overseen the clinical tests on prisoners carried out by R. Eugene Dyer, who recruited Shannon to NIH as associate director of the Heart Institute in charge of research and who was Shannon's predecessor as NIH director.) Shannon was tall, reticent, a bit flat on first impression, and eventually a whiz at building programs and policies at NIH. Among his first orders of business was reinventing Guinea Pig Units in the cold war political climate.

The great virtue of religious objectors was that they were healthy, pliant, and cheap. Thus, two days before Christmas 1952, the executive secretary of the National Service Board for Religious Objectors, A. S. Curry, came to NIH's Building 1 to start negotiations for a formal program that would bring men drafted for the Korean War to the Clinical Center to be studied.[45] Shannon had been promoted to associate director of all of NIH earlier that year, and he did most of the talking for the agency. A dozen NIH clinical and administrative leaders listened in. Irving Ladimer, from Research Planning, was among this group. Ladimer later drafted policies for the Normal Volunteer Patient Program and was on the three-man committee that crafted the group-consideration guidelines. Also at the table was Dr. Donald Whedon, whose protocol was the NIH test case for the Normals program.[46] Dr. Russell Wilder was disappointed to have to miss this important meeting to set up the Normals program: he had been appointed a few months earlier to lead the small committee to write what later became the group-consideration guidelines.

The program seemed to fit the needs of both the Clinical Center and the National Service Board for Religious Objectors, and so the specifics were locked into place over the next year. Carl was in fact a Mennonite drafted to serve in the Korean War. NIH researchers imagined that the beliefs of his "religious sect," implied Carl had "very firm beliefs and convictions" against "either wearing the uniform or carrying a gun." Carl's feelings about his service at the Clinical Center show how the interests of his church and of NIH converged both in the Normals program and in the flesh and blood of people like him. Personally, Carl felt "great conflict over his religious beliefs," and his medical chart recorded:

> [He] accepted service as a conscientious objector to please his family and church congregation rather than joining the Army or Air Force to please himself. [He has the] feeling that he is "against a stone wall" and doesn't know which way to turn; his church congregation has no interest in him and that "people have turned their backs on him"; he is a failure, unworthy and has stood about all he can bear. . . . He expressed guilt over dancing and drinking a few beers several years ago, over watching TV and attending movies here, and that his church teaches that they are wrong but he cannot feel that they are wrong for him.[47]

The strong religious community nonetheless aided Shannon in his negotiations with the National Service Board for Religious Objectors. He expected that researchers would need healthy subjects for a few weeks or months at a time; Curry pressed for more open-ended stays, since he was trying to fill service assignments that spanned years. They agreed on flexible stays, so long as the men were under no illusion that NIH would hire Normals for permanent jobs.

From his side of the bargaining table, Curry cautioned researchers that religious objectors might choose more heroic assignments than living in a hospital. But, more optimistically, he knew of several hundred men in the area who needed placements. The rhetoric of valor permeated efforts to recruit Normals, in part because the assignment was seen by many people as an unpatriotic cop-out for America's boys. Sick patients, for instance, occasionally refused to share rooms with Normals. Even clinicians, most of whom had served in the war as officers, had to be reminded when dealing with the pacifists, "Although these are not our convictions, it is our position to respect these beliefs of theirs insofar as it is possible for [researchers] to do it, as one human being to another."[48] Researchers who scorned the beliefs of conscientious objectors may have, nonetheless, appreciated that the objectors enabled their studies to go forward. And many Americans did feel that serving science as a research subject was a noble sacrifice, if not the same as seeing battle. Citizens pleaded to be subjects in nuclear-weapons tests in the South Pacific after the war, and an exclusive fraternal organization, called the Guinea Pig Society, began around this time.[49]

Given their interests, NIH leaders encouraged the heroic slant. One of Carl's contemporaries, a twenty-six-year-old farmer from Idaho, consented to have his left thigh opened up and a piece of muscle removed for lab study. When he returned to Idaho, he received a certificate from the director of the Clinical Center "attesting to the contribution" he had made "to the advancement of medicine and of man's knowledge of himself." He was informed, "Your voluntary participation in medical research studies at the National Institutes of Health was an unselfish contribution to mankind everywhere, and for all time to come." Regardless of how the young farmer felt about having a leg operation cast in this light—proud, skeptical, mystified?—it would seem that the researchers held their own work in high esteem.[50]

For the time being, the appeal to national sacrifice allowed Shannon to drive a hard financial bargain with Curry. Shannon had assumed NIH could get the men at low cost, as he had done in World War II. For the church leaders, one of the harsh lessons of the previous program was that coordinating placements was costly for the organizations and serving without pay had left men destitute. The only compensation the men received for their work during World War II was the pleasure of not being imprisoned for draft-dodging. This was one feature of the program Curry was keen to change. Eventually, Shannon and Curry agreed that NIH would "'purchase' services from the organizations on a man-month basis," using the pay scale set up for a program at the University of Michigan. The church organizations would give the men a small stipend after taking an administrative fee for placing them.[51] When Normals came to the Clinical Center, starting in 1954, the NIH paid sponsor organizations around $100 per month per head, $15 of which went to the Normal control. (The men's stipend would be worth about $150 in 2010.) Of course, there were small additional costs to NIH. The healthy patients had to be fed—by all accounts the food from the Clinical Center kitchen was quite tasty, and all the more delectable when a healthy patient was coming off a restricted diet. Their clothes and linens were washed in the industrial laundry in the basement, and just to be on the safe side in this unprecedented arrangement, NIH paid a bit extra so that churches could buy liability insurance for the first Normal controls recruited through the organizations.[52] All told, NIH reported that it cost a mere $3.85 per day to keep a Normal at the Clinical Center. It is not clear whether the agency was more pleased by the bargain or by the precision with which they had calculated the expense.[53]

In 1953 researchers were eager to start their studies with healthy patients and awaited news about whether the Normal Volunteer Patient Program would be allowed. It was a relatively long wait, because after Shannon signed off on the program that he had brokered, the proposal went to the surgeon general for approval, and then on to the secretary of the Department of Health, Education, and Welfare because of its serious "public relations implications."[54] A few weeks later, NIH employees learned of the program's approval in a memo restricted from general release. It explained, "Except for dietary restrictions and some controlled physical activity, there will be no risk or inconvenience" and said that the projects would be reviewed and approved in advance by the Medical Board. Reading on, NIH employees may have been puzzled to learn that Mennonite and Brethren volunteers were ideal subjects precisely because of their "intelligent acceptance of possible hazard and inconvenience."[55]

Once the legal infrastructure was in place, though, NIH administrators immediately opened the Normals program to bring in citizens who had no obligation to the government. In 1954 NIH arranged to bring in any members of peace churches, not only conscientious objectors. Around the age of twenty, many young adults in these churches left their communities for a year of service. Researchers thought there was no better place than the Clinical Center to witness the teachings of Jesus, and they were frankly puzzled why they didn't "get more of these young people."[56] The staff members were eager to solve this riddle, and when they asked Normals, they learned that young Christians had expected that by witnessing in a hospital they would spend more time comforting sick patients and less time serving as healthy patients themselves. Fewer religious volunteers were serving by 1960, after a final rally in which a motorcade delivered fifty-nine Brethren and Mennonite college students to the Clinical Center at a time when the total hospital occupancy hovered around 60 percent with roughly three hundred full beds. Cuing recruits to see the financial, educational, and religious benefits, NIH encouraged Normals toward the hospital with the slogan "earn, learn, and serve."[57] NIH continued in vain to recruit from the church organizations that had first structured the program, but they could not gloss over the disappointment that lingered for church leaders over the experiences of early volunteers.

Energized to fill the gap left by church volunteers on top of the growing demand for healthy patients from researchers, NIH administrators soon

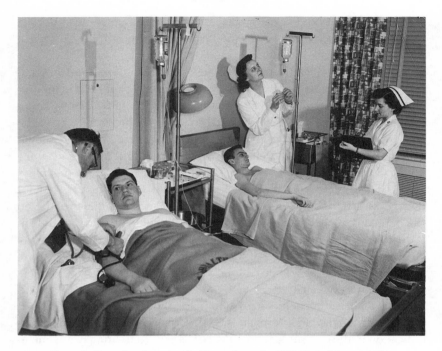

Figure 5. Normal patients enrolled in studies at the NIH Clinical Center, 1958.
Courtesy of the Mennonite Church USA.

struck deals to get Normal controls from civic organizations, from the Bureau of Prisons, and from two small cities (Johnston, Pennsylvania, and Beckley, West Virginia) that had experienced economic downturns. The only requirements were that the men have their sanity and all of their appendages intact. Conscripts and prisoners aside, the saving grace of the Normals program was college students. The activist-minded students had been drawn by the proximity to Washington's political scene, especially during Vietnam protests and civil rights rallies in the mid-1960s. These unshaven, sandal-wearing students were a persistent source of annoyance for the program coordinator, Delbert Nye, and he was pleased to report in 1966 that the men were "better barbered," even if more women were wearing shorts and jeans.[58] Excluding prisoners, by the 1970s, around 90 percent of Normals were college students, many of whom came during summer break.[59] Some students were motivated by being able to add NIH job experience to their resumes and medical school applications as the agency's prestige grew. What researchers at the Clinical Center came to know about the human body from their research during this period was, more precisely, known about young white middle-class Americans aspiring for great careers and for a better political future.

Still, the program that enabled research on healthy Americans at the Clinical Center in the first place had started under political circumstances quite different from those marked by the civil rights agenda that were familiar to 1970s citizens (and research participants). In 1954, one of the

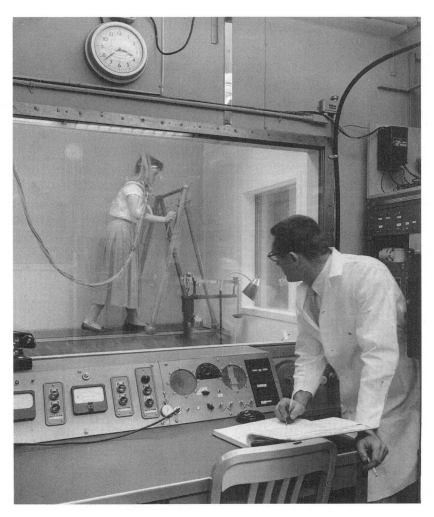

Figure 6. Mennonite woman in a respiration helmet for a metabolism study at the Clinical Center; a researcher (smoking) observes, 1958. Courtesy of the Mennonite Church USA.

last points of negotiation with church groups concerned the name of the program. NIH leaders worked to round off the coarse edges of the wartime Guinea Pig Units for the program's peacetime incarnation with civilians. "As a special favor, if you can possibly avoid using the 'guinea pig' label, please do so," religious groups were requested. "There is a Buchenwald connotation in this phrase which is totally false, and we are doing everything possible to discourage it."[60]

The Wilder Committee

This is how, in the autumn of 1954, Carl Zimmerman came to receive a letter at his home in rural Pennsylvania that precipitated his move to the Clinical Center. At the time, Carl was working as a farmhand for his family's small dairy after getting fired from his job as a local garbage collector.[61] The letter was from the Selective Service, and it told Carl to report to his new job as a soldier in the U.S. military. Carl made the half-day drive south into Maryland so he could serve out his tour of duty with the Public Health Service as a conscientious objector to the Korean War.

Generally speaking, the immediate post–World War II years were a high point in popular support for biomedical research and the authority of science. Thousands of Washingtonians visited the Clinical Center to tour the labs, see feature films, and attend public lectures; this was part of a concerted "public relations campaign" imagined years earlier to "sell" the hospital to Americans and also to leave members of Congress with the impression that the taxpayers were sold on it.[62]

This bit of dazzle seemed in order because there were several factions that resisted federal funding of research in the years leading up to the Clinical Center opening. Critics charged that government sponsorship of science would shape research results in unfavorable ways—a concern, incidentally, that is reiterated whenever patterns of patronage change, whether from philanthropies to the government during the mid-twentieth century or from the government to private industry, more recently.[63] In the early 1950s, the enthusiasm of members of Congress for health-related research was just beginning to grow.[64] But publicly sponsored research was suspect because of its allegedly protocommunist commitment to socialized medicine.[65] In addition, some critics took issue with the NIH's "categorical approach," in which research was organized around specific diseases, such as heart disease, cancer, and mental illness. Among university-based researchers, the problem was not with government funding of research per se, but rather with the requirement that researchers hitch themselves to a specific research mission at NIH to receive federal money for studies at their home institutions. The American Medical Association led the charge against government-sponsored medicine in the interest of its members. It was a common refrain in postwar science-policy circles: science, like capitalism, and like democracy itself, was diminished, not enhanced, by heavy-handed federal direction.[66]

For these critics, the plan of building a government-owned and government-operated research hospital would be a particularly egregious case of state intrusion into science. University researchers felt that NIH should continue to use public money to award grants (i.e., to fund them, the university researchers) rather than to take on clinical research within the federal bureaucracy. Many NIH scientists left the agency in protest of the plan to build the Clinical Center, and Clinical Center leaders saw themselves competing for talent against not only universities but also "progressive private industry." Indeed, many of the forward-thinking hiring policies at NIH—hiring Jews, women, and married couples—were in fact recruiting tools. If they could not offer extravagant pay and total freedom, NIH leaders felt it was essential that they promise potential hires other resources they needed, including clinical materials such as human subjects, with as much free rein as they could let out.[67]

When the senior scientists who made up the NIH Medical Board planned for the Clinical Center opening, they knew that even if their practices were formally unregulated according to the familiar rhetoric of scientific freedom, they would nonetheless be closely watched to make sure they were compassionate investigators and good Americans. The target of any formal research guidelines—or, more to the point, the news that there were research guidelines at the Clinical Center—included potential patient-recruits such as Carl, public onlookers such as the locals who would be touring the hospital as part of the NIH public relations campaign, and, as always, members of Congress with money to give and to take away.

Although the spectacle of responsibility was important, NIH leaders also wanted to reduce the actual chances of a research accident that would prompt bad press, congressional scrutiny, or a lawsuit. At the Clinical Center, problems would not arise from devious researchers, they assured themselves, but from a lack of communication and coordination between the separate institutes. Normals posed a special problem. Healthy patients were not proprietary, and they were very valuable clinical material. Researchers anticipated using a Normal in more than one study at a time, passing them from study to study, institute to institute. For example, Carl was admitted to the National Heart Institute but was used in studies from at least three institutes before he left.[68] Greater efficiency was a goal often articulated and rarely achieved at the Clinical Center. But it was in the spirit of efficiency that administrators circulated lists of patients and their diagnoses to alert researchers of available "clinical materials." It was not until 1957, the year Carl left the Clinical Center, that Shannon, by then NIH director, imposed a record-based system for tracking the studies in which Normals were enrolled.

Under the political scrutiny of the early 1950s, NIH leaders felt it was crucial to figure out how to achieve their primary and pragmatic goal, which was to build a bulwark against legal action. In the words of clinical directors from 1952, research guidelines would serve "as a counter-balance and check to protect not only the patient but the Institute involved and the Clinical Center as a whole."[69] Early NIH leaders tried to strike a sensitive balance. They claimed to potential hires that researchers would enjoy research with few restrictions at the Clinical Center. They also tried to show they placed responsible limits on research to satisfy federal lawyers and appropriations committees on Capitol Hill.

The Wilder Committee invented the solution. In the autumn of 1951, Dr. Russell Wilder learned he was to lead "a small task force," which came to be known as the Wilder Committee, to deal with questions about "policies of the NIH having to do with studies and investigations on human subjects."[70] Wilder was director of the National Institute of Arthritis and Metabolic Diseases (today called the National Institute of Diabetes and Digestive and Kidney Disorders). Among scientists, Wilder came to be best known for his research on nutrition and food rationing. Among Normals he was distinguished for the culinary abomination they consumed while on one of his studies. In addition, though Carl may not have known it, Wilder's nutrition research was to blame for nurses' enduring fascination with his stool samples. In any event, in 1951 Wilder learned that Irving Ladimer would be the executive secretary for his new administrative task and that Dr. G. Burroughs "Bo" Mider would be his compatriot clinician.

The Wilder Committee drafted policies for the Clinical Center on the use of human subjects. This assignment came from Norman Topping, a legend on the old softball field where the Clinical Center was now being built and also director of intramural research at NIH. (Recall that the Intramural Program is the research program internal to NIH that included the Clinical Center; the Extramural Program funds research at other research locations, such as hospitals and universities.) Topping had recently returned from a 1951 speaking tour of the leading medical schools and the American Medical Association headquarters in Chicago. His mission was to assure medical researchers that government science, such as the work that researchers would be doing at the Clinical Center, did not require subservience to politicians, administrators, and bureaucrats. Scientific freedom was the aspiration of the day, and Topping's job had been to explain how NIH ensured that decisions were made by scientists, for scientists, for the betterment of science.[71]

The Wilder Committee is best thought of as a subset of three men within an already close-knit group of Clinical Center leaders, collectively known as the Medical Board. Meeting for the first time in 1952, the Medical Board was the small and powerful committee charged with setting common policies that all the institutes would follow when the Clinical Center opened in 1953. The board comprised the director of the Clinical Center, each of the institutes' clinical directors, and six other scientists whom they would choose.[72] Drs. Wilder and Mider were members of the Medical Board in the early 1950s, and Irving Ladimer frequently attended meetings. The Wilder Committee members were thus sympathetic to the needs of clinical researchers, and they would write the raw proposals that the full Medical Board molded into livable policy to guide research on sick and healthy patients. As Mider understood their job, the three men were to study "the ethical and medicolegal aspects of the forthcoming clinical research program."[73] A decade later, Mider recalled that the committee was asked to draft a policy because NIH leaders worried that work inside the publicly funded center "would be open to inspection by all" and that researchers would be "looked at intensely and probably by unfriendly eyes." The Wilder Committee was to deal with the fact that "NIH was going to be doing clinical research in a goldfish bowl."[74]

With calls for legal protection on the one hand and for unfettered research on the other, it was unclear what the Wilder Committee was to do. Adopting an ethics code would have been typical for an organization in need of a research ethics policy in the 1950s, since expert group decision making was not an obvious way to oversee human-subjects research at the time. Had Carl gone into the army when he was drafted, as he had wished, military researchers would have assured his protection as a research participant using the language of the 1947 Nuremberg Code, which privileged the good judgment of the morally upstanding (read *democratic*) doctor.[75] The U.S. Department of Defense adopted the Nuremberg Code to guide field research on soldiers in 1953, the same year that NIH adopted group-consideration guidelines. NIH clinicians would have been aware of the adoption of the

Nuremberg Code in the armed forces, even though the policy was confidential at the time.[76] NIH scientists talked regularly with other military officers—the Public Health Service was still part of the Federal Security Agency until 1953—at Washington science venues such as Atomic Energy Commission meetings. In Bethesda, NIH scientists often rolled down their shirtsleeves to take lunch with navy scientists at the Officers' Club across the street at the Naval Medical Center.[77] It was de rigueur to say that any policy on the treatment of human subjects was modeled, in spirit, on the Nuremberg Code. NIH leaders asserted this, as well, but what the code represented to them in the 1950s differs from twenty-first-century understandings. At NIH, for example, it was the pinnacle of research ethics to state that studies followed the Nuremberg Code's precept that no experiment should be done in which the researchers believed subjects could die or be disabled—unless, that is, "the experimentalist physician also serves as subject."[78] Hand-waving aside, researchers generally regarded the Nuremberg Code as a set of principles appropriate for moral monsters, not for democratically minded American physicians.[79]

The Code of Ethics of the American Medical Association might have been a viable alternative, but NIH leaders believed it addressed research on sick patients exclusively. Ladimer, for one, found the AMA code of ethics silent on the newest and most exciting topic of research: studies on Normals. "Physicians do not ordinarily practice on normal people," Ladimer pointed out to his audience at the AMA annual meeting in 1955. "One is therefore concerned with a distinct type of endeavor. The law has not set out permissible limits for this field as it has for medical practice."[80] There was something different about doing research on healthy citizens in hospitals, Ladimer felt, something that was not articulated in codes of medical ethics.

Outside observers agreed. Clinicians had long relied on the convenient idiom of the doctor-patient relationship that was embedded in codes of medical ethics. It allowed them to retain authority and discretion in clinical decision making. Out of either habit or conviction, NIH clinicians at times slipped into the analogy, describing healthy patients as comparable to sick patients in their relationships with researchers. During a 1954 meeting after the first batch of Normals had arrived in Bethesda, for example, clinicians made this view clear to A. S. Curry, who was now the Mennonite volunteer coordinator after having brokered the deal with NIH to start the Normals program for religious objectors, including Carl. During the meeting, Curry got the sense that "doctors felt it was impossible to explain experiments to the subjects and he got the feeling that they [didn't] want to be bothered with questions by the 'patients.'" Curry added, "It was brought out in the interview many times that the basic relationship is that of <u>doctor-patient</u> and that the doctor in charge of the patient has full supervision over all that he does. One can understand why a 'wide awake,' healthy volunteer would be more inquiring and want to know more about what is going on than a very sick patient who has no interest in the scientific aspect of the work."[81] Even when researchers themselves felt the analogy was not apt, they repeated the familiar rhetoric in part because, even though the characteristics of the patients had changed, privileging the good judgment of scientists continued to make sense to them at a time when they considered themselves to be morally exceptional.[82]

As a matter of local politics, members of the Medical Board were also hesitant to adopt an ethics code because they did not want to privilege one institute at the Clinical Center over another. One of the many legacies of World War II for physicians and scientists was that research areas splintered into increasingly fine, self-referential areas of specialization. At NIH, clinicians shared standards—both formal and conventional—with researchers from their home institutes. They only shared standards with researchers in other institutes and specialties, they felt, in the loosest sense. NIH planners, who likewise felt allegiances to their own kind, built these local cultures into the Clinical Center. Members of the Medical Board, representing all of the different institutes, worked toward the common purpose of insulating researchers in one institute from impositions of the other institutes. During the planning stages of the hospital, for example, the six men in charge of their institutes' interests in the Clinical Center decided to duplicate some services and staff pools inside the building, rather than to have common resources. Tellingly, they imagined the Clinical Center building as several autonomous hospitals.[83]

Similarly, members of the Medical Board did not want researchers in their home institutes beholden to published ethics codes or informal moralities that had originated in other fields. Psychiatrists should not be constrained by the standards of dentists, they agreed. In setting research guidelines, in particular, Medical Board members were keen to avoid situations in which "certain parts of the document suited the plans of some institutes but not of others." In place of rigidity and uniformity, they aspired to be "more flexible in order to accommodate the differences."[84] Indeed, investigators were primed to develop distinctive research practices within each institute, because the administrative structure of NIH from its inception was heavily decentralized, leaving programs and procedures—with the exception of the Clinical Center effort—to the will of each institute director.

Adding to the opposition to an ethics code, NIH lawyers pressed for a policy beyond the sacred doctor-patient relationship. Edward Rourke was legal counsel to the Clinical Center through the 1950s and 1960s, a career that spans decades and the next two chapters. On this early issue, Rourke's concern was that ethics codes were specific to professions, not to places. A researcher, by virtue of his professional training, was imagined to have the sound judgment that made his actions ethical. Violations raised questions not about the site where the research was done, but about the authenticity of the professional—in other words, whether the researcher was, in fact, a well-trained member of the profession or a quack. Ethics codes did not locate individual researchers within buildings, but within imagined moral communities of fellow practitioners. The ideal alternative, in the eyes of lawyers in the Office of General Counsel, was the use of standardized, signed "consent" or "release" forms.[85] Rourke pressed this position later in the 1950s and was later disappointed with researchers' intransigence regarding consent forms. On the immediate question of ethics policy, though, Rourke and the Office of General Counsel aimed to protect NIH, brick and mortar.

Inventing Group Consideration

In 1952 and 1953, as the facility's opening date drew near, researchers still had the authority to write the policies that would bind them. The Medical Board and the Wilder Committee, in particular, felt strained by the limits of codes of ethics. Shannon, from his post as associate director of NIH at this time, encouraged his subordinates to create a procedure for expert review to manage this seeming impasse.[86] They wanted a policy but did not want an ethics code. Shannon imagined a policy for the entire Clinical Center that accommodated local practices of the institutes cordoned within it, a policy that respected clinicians' bedside authority even over patients who did not fit the traditional mold. Heeding Shannon's advice, the Wilder Committee circumvented the problems of physical and professional balkanization inside the Clinical Center by inventing a procedure enacted by an expert group, rather than writing a set of rules for institutes to share.

Group consideration would work like this: As a first tier of review, researchers talked about studies on sick patients during ward rounds, which was when members of an institute walked through the hospital rooms discussing cases. The 1953 group-consideration guidelines also specified, however, that if scientists had special worries that they could not settle with their institute colleagues, they should contact the Medical Board's Clinical Research Committee (CRC). This committee, made up of a subset of board members, was created solely to offer a second tier of review by experts uninvolved in investigators' research. As the Medical Board explained, the Clinical Research Committee would field "novel questions or issues of wide significance" from the categorical institutes and forward its recommendations for a given protocol to the director of NIH for approval.[87] In extreme circumstances, protocols indicating that a policy change was in order would get forwarded to the third level of review, which was a step higher in the Public Health Service chain of command: the surgeon general and his advisers. Although the Medical Board made the review system elective in most cases, the second layer of review was compulsory for research on subjects involving "unusual hazard."[88]

In addition, all studies on Normal patients were supposed to go through the CRC.[89] During the 1950s, around 90 percent of the studies that the CRC reviewed were studies on Normals. The other 10 percent were very risky studies on sick people. For example, in the committee's first year, thirty-four studies were approved through group consideration, all but two of which were for Normals. In 1958 the CRC approved all thirty-seven studies it reviewed, and all but one of them were on Normals.[90] As their meeting records show, the beauty of the practice was that they were able to hold fast to the tradition of deferring to doctors' good judgment, and at the same time they created evidence that the decision was not made solely by an individual doctor but by a group of doctors instead.

It was a capacious policy organized around professional discretion, but it also created a paper trail of conversation. Case in point: in reviewing one infectious-disease study submitted by Dr. Vernon Knight (an important figure in chapter 6) the committee recorded that they were "relying on the good judgment of Dr. Knight and his colleagues and their advice to the Committee that this is a relatively minor illness."[91] The fact that we have a record of the discussion suggests the importance of group considerations in documenting that a consensual decision was made. By constituting an expert group's decision as, by definition, the proper way to proceed, group-consideration guidelines allowed tremendous flexibility for clinical researchers and allowed legal protection for the place itself, or so they hoped.

This literal step, from the Clinical Center ward to the conference room, split apart a medico-ethical-legal practice that had traditionally been all one piece. This move, for better or worse, encouraged researchers to make a conceptual distinction between science and ethics. They were able to conceptualize and talk about the ward as the place where they did science and the conference room as the place where they worried about ethics and legalities.

In short, Clinical Center leaders created a policy that protected the place, and not a policy focused on the individual researcher. They aimed to coordinate activities inside the hospital, particularly with Normals, and group consideration served this purpose well. Group consideration was a novel form of ethics decision making that invested moral authority in the group itself. No one person—neither clinician, nor patient, nor supervisor—had the sole power to decide whether research could proceed. Tellingly, when the Medical Board formally adopted group consideration as policy in 1953, its members decided to distribute copies of the policy via the institutes, rather than sending a copy to everyone in the Clinical Center, because they "recognized that some interpretation of the document [would] be necessary."[92] They felt that this interpretation should occur among members of the same institute. The great advantage of the group-consideration procedure was that it gave researchers who were all within one building the ability to use one decision-making method that could nonetheless accommodate different institutes.

In the period when the Clinical Center opened, a few other texts, such as the Nuremberg Code and the Code of Ethics of the American Medical Association (two documents that, not coincidentally, were very similar), also prescribed how investigators should interact with their research subjects. What was unusual about the Clinical Center's group-consideration guidelines was that they recommended that in certain circumstances a group of researchers uninvolved in the study weigh in on the question of whether their colleagues had planned appropriately to protect their research participants. By extension the group also considered the legal integrity and reputation of the facility in which they all worked. The four-page document laying out the group-consideration guidelines marks the move away from deference to investigators' personal discretion and toward deference to committee procedures in decisions about the treatment of research participants.

Conclusion: An Ethics of Place

The NIH Clinical Center opened in July 1953, and it was in planning for this new research facility that its Medical Board wrote the group-consideration guidelines, officially called "Group Consideration of Clinical Research Procedures Deviating from Accepted Medical Practice or Involving Unusual Hazard." Inventing the practice of group consideration it created a procedure in which a committee uninvolved in the research would judge whether an investigator had planned to protect his human subjects. Group consideration did not have a long tradition in clinical research prior to 1953. To be sure, scientists in earlier periods sorted out quandaries by talking with each other and by watching other scientists in their midst. Through these tacit practices, communities of scientists developed what Sydney Halpern has called "indigenous moralities," the local sensibilities about the boundaries of acceptable research.[93] The men who came up with rules for research at the Clinical Center observed that other "responsible research organizations" had "generally adopted practices and procedures which insure high standards of professional, legal, and moral conduct," but that these were "not usually written."[94] Like their contemporaries, NIH researchers' first instinct was that no rules needed to be written down. Nonetheless, in November 1953, the surgeon general of the Public Health Service formally endorsed group consideration as the practice that would ensure upstanding research at the NIH Clinical Center.

The theory behind the 1953 group-consideration guidelines was that the procedure they outlined would accommodate conflicting preferences for broad oversight and professional autonomy, universal ideals and local practices, while allowing some semblance of rules to encase the publicly funded facility. Group consideration was novel in that it required prior deliberation—intervention before investigators could make potential misjudgments. New assumptions about researchers were also built into the procedure: board members felt that even the brightest scientists had some measure of moral fallibility and that groups of scientists deliberating together could make better judgments than individuals in lone reflection. Despite these innovations, group consideration also reinforced many of the assumptions familiar in contemporary arguments supporting investigators' discretion in the treatment of research participants. By locating moral authority in the process of group consideration, sick and healthy patients were kept from making decisions about their research fate. Implicit in group consideration was the belief that researchers should still participate in the evaluation of their own studies, but that other people—a group of expert colleagues—had a greater claim to sound moral judgment. Thus, while a researcher's intimacy with his own study was to blame for his occasionally distorted view of its importance and its low risks, social and scientific closeness was precisely what gave his colleagues a privileged perspective in judging the ethical acceptability of his research. Decades later, researchers were removed from review meetings because of concerns over conflict of interest. This is one of the ironies of expert group review: those who know the most about studies are also presumed to have the greatest stake in the outcome—and thus the most distorted opinions. As chapter 1 documents, the unintuitive ways in which NIH created and enforced ethics practices reverberate in present-day IRB meetings.

It can be tempting to look at what is today a large government organization and assume that any question was destined to be answered with the suggestion that a committee be appointed. In the early 1950s, however, this was far from obvious at NIH. Certainly, group consideration resonated with routines familiar to NIH researchers: ward rounds and animal-use committees, for example.[95] But research was sacred territory, and Clinical Center leaders railed against any perceived incursions into scientists' autonomous decision making. This position served their personal interests as researchers, no doubt, but it also mapped onto scientists' insistence at the time that NIH had to ward off any suggestion that the government was inhibiting the free practice of science.

Most profoundly, a new kind of patient—the healthy patient—came into existence at the Clinical Center. Through the Normal Volunteer Patient Program, healthy American civilians came to live at the hospital. In the planning stages, the program was advocated as a patriotic alternative for conscientious objectors to the Korean War, but after 1954 the Normals program never depended on the draft again. Through the rest of the decade, NIH leaders promoted the logic of what we now call nontherapeutic research for citizen-subjects, defined in their words as "acts conducted in the name of research [that] do not necessarily imply immediate benefit to the subject."[96] The aim of medical intervention could be the greater good of science, not the improvement of a person's health, whether sick or healthy.

The practice of group consideration and the Normals program shaped and sustained each other. The two innovations—healthy patients and group review—informed each other deeply because in the early 1950s, the NIH Clinical Center was being built on uncertain political ground. Even after Congress had appropriated funds for the facility, its future looked dim during several moments of political crisis in the early 1950s. Rules for patient care were part of a broader effort to steel the Clinical Center against critics and intruders imagined to be inevitable in a public research hospital. To this end, Clinical Center leaders aspired to coordinate the research that would take place inside the building—for the integrity of their research, the legal protection of NIH, and the physical protection of subjects. But the categorical institutes that would be sharing the hospital were highly balkanized, and they were to be spread across a sprawling fourteen-story building.

The virtue of group consideration, to members of the Medical Board in 1953, was that it could accommodate the tremendous incoherence of the institutes and retain the professional discretion researchers had traditionally enjoyed. An expert group would have the discretion to recognize different standards for different institutes, to show deference to researchers as circumstances seemed to merit, and to encourage flexible consent proce-dures for different kinds of patients—another tricky problem, as chapter 5 shows. Group review appeased problems of pride and practicality among researchers who were poorly organized to share resources, especially healthy patients like Carl.

As a consequence, NIH created a policy that bound the Clinical Center as a place. NIH leaders wrote the policy to suit the distinctive arrangement of the Clinical Center in the early 1950s. In the past, ethics codes had com-monly been used to defend members of a profession, such as surgeons, physicians, anthropologists, or nurses and to police professional bound-aries. NIH leaders, by contrast, created a formal legitimate alternative to profession-based ethics. It was a workable arrangement for the legal, intel-lectual, and physical circumstances of the Clinical Center in the 1950s. The guidelines protected the site primarily, and the scientists and subjects inside it coincidentally.

This was the same set of circumstances that Carl, ultimately, did not want to forgo. Twenty-four months was the span of his debt to his country, and Carl's obligation was paid in full by December 1956, which left him free to go. But it was a cold winter, and returning to labor on his family's farm did not appeal. Although he complained about the routines, the restrictions, the nurses, and the food, he had started to take comfort in them after two years. As they accrued, the rituals showed Carl that, perhaps for the first time in his life, he had a place. And so this difficult patient begged to stay. Dr. Fredrickson, for one, was delighted to let Carl stay through the new year. Fredrickson had a study in mind for which he needed Normal controls. So on his penultimate day at the Clinical Center, Carl was injected with human blood serum that was tagged with radioactive carbon, observed overnight, and discharged the next morning. Group review made this research on Carl possible. And group review not only survived out of inertia but thrived into the 1960s as clinicians attributed ever more virtues to the practice in defense of professional discretion.

FIVE

The Many Forms of Consent

There have been some rather naïve discussions in the literature on the question of oral or written, formal or informal, expressed or implied types [of consent]. I will say flatly (as I have said very frequently) that consent does not become any better, does not become any more legal, because it is written. . . . For many purposes it may be desirable not to wave papers around and make it look like a real estate transaction or a death notice. There are other ways to get well-documented consent. Whatever is done, however, certainly must be included and incorporated in any record.

—Irving Ladimer, November 12, 1964

Proof of Consent, 1953–1963

Sarah Isaac had a talent for keeping track of things. She kept such good records of her stay at the Clinical Center that doctors cited her data when writing notes in her chart: "According to the patient's count (and she kept careful records) she had 458 hours with Dr. Day." Her record-keeping required a certain discipline, not to mention literacy and perceptual acuity. Sarah had "a brilliant mind, an overwhelming sensitivity, not only directed inward, but toward the grasp of phenomenon [sic] beyond her."[1]

With her knack for record-keeping and her ability to express her feelings, Sarah came into her own in the late 1950s as a Normal control for Charles Savage's research on an experimental drug that had been created only a decade earlier: LSD.[2] After a year on several other wards for studies of the thyroid and of new steroids, Sarah moved to the 3-West nursing ward as the only person in the control arm of Dr. Savage's studies that examined whether LSD helped schizophrenics in psychotherapy. Sarah was given the

drug between one and four times per week while she lived alongside traditional patients enrolled in the research.

We know a surprising amount about what Sarah Isaac felt while she was
at the Clinical Center in the mid-1950s. Her record-keeping bent made her
"an utterly fascinating patient," a mutual enchantment that doctors at the
Clinical Center sustained for three and a half years. During this time, researchers asked her to keep a journal about how she felt on LSD. Sarah also
wrote reproachful notes to nurses and long letters—some days affectionate,
other days hostile—to doctors and social workers.[3] "She could be utterly
engaging, witty, charming and pretty, or cunning and delicately hostile, subtly manipulative and ugly," one psychiatrist recorded. "The latter state was
usually in response to a situation in which the patient felt degraded and her
action was in the direction of lowering the esteem of the other and this was
frequently quite successful."[4] Yet it is hard to know what Sarah and the doctors actually said to each other.

Conversations between researchers and research subjects were ephemeral
during the 1950s and 1960s. Those that took place in the Clinical Center
vanished in the hospital wards, and so we know only what Sarah and NIH
employees committed to paper. Hospital rooms before the 1970s have been
portrayed as silent worlds, in the memorable phrase of physician, ethicist,
and historian Jay Katz.[5] In this silent world, doctors did too many things
without telling others and spoke too little about their uncertainties. Yet it is
worth remembering that not everything that was spoken was written down
in ways considered conventional by present-day legal and scientific standards. This fact points to the crux of the debate in the late 1950s and early
1960s over what counted as proof of consent and, more important, who
got to define it.

This chapter explores debates between NIH researchers and lawyers
about how to document subjects' consent. By the 1950s, there was no debate
whether researchers needed to get consent. The controversies were about
how to *prove* that researchers had "gotten" this thing—namely, acknowl-
edgment that people knew they were being studied—a legal right recently
brought into being in the postwar public consciousness.[6] At NIH during the
1950s and 1960s, researchers and lawyers battled over what would constitute evidence that subjects had been asked and had agreed to be studied and
that consent, when given, was genuine. As a consequence of these debates,
researchers invested the practice of group review with even more virtue and
authority. This decision-making method allowed researchers to hold on to
expert discretion in deciding what counted as evidence of consent, rather
than to adopt a standardized, form-based consent policy.

By the time the surgeon general imposed the institutional review system on universities, hospitals, and other research organizations in 1966, scientists at NIH had systematically, if begrudgingly, started to collect signed forms as evidence of consent from sick patients. As for healthy patients, the 1962 amendments to the Food and Drug Act had required researchers to collect signatures on consent forms for trials of new, experimental drugs, many of which were under study at the Clinical Center.[7] In practice, however, NIH researchers occasionally fell short, which is surprising only if we believe the rhetoric that the NIH researchers were demigods, not mortal like the rest of us. More interestingly, many Clinical Center researchers intentionally avoided collecting signed forms from Normal controls if such forms were not required, into the early 1960s. Researchers felt that there were other adequate ways of documenting healthy patients' consent, for example, by making notes in their medical records. At the Clinical Center, researchers argued that the Medical Board's Clinical Research Committee had the authority to define adequate proof of consent and that there should not be one standard policy for sick and healthy patients, nor for all studies across institutes. Researchers, in other words, argued for discretion and for their own authority to decide on a case-by-case basis what counted as adequate proof of consent.

As important as they were, the 1962 Drug Amendments did not require proof of written consent for all studies on healthy people. Unlike human-subjects regulations today, the Drug Amendments bound a type of research (i.e., drug trials), not a population of research subjects (for example, prisoners). This is why NIH director James Shannon saw no consistent method of proving consent within the Clinical Center at the time. Although some institutes used signed forms rigorously, if Shannon had walked the wards of his own National Heart Institute in 1965, he would have found a different set of consent practices. Although formal policy at the Clinical Center as of 1958 stated that researchers should collect signed forms from Normals, Dr. Robert Berliner, the director of the National Heart Institute, did not require researchers to collect signed consent documents either from sick patients or from Normal controls.[8] And among institutes within the Clinical Center that did use a standard form, one institute's form differed from another's. NIH lawyers in the Office of General Counsel certainly felt that proof of consent on paper was strongest legally. The debate over documenting consent was protracted because it was an open question as to what would hold up in court. Since clinical research on healthy people was new, lawsuits were likewise unprecedented. In the debate over evidence of consent at the Clinical Center during the late 1950s and early 1960s, NIH researchers generally worked to keep their traditional authority and discretion, and law-yers erred on the side of legal caution.

For NIH researchers, the Medical Board's Clinical Research Committee was indispensible. Researchers argued that there were multiple valid ways to create evidence of consent and that the appropriate method of document-ing consent in a given case would be best determined by a group of experts. This chapter shows that the group-review model that Clinical Center leaders created in the early 1950s became ingrained as part of hospital routine dur-ing the late 1950s and early 1960s because it was the mechanism through which NIH researchers defined *how* human subjects' consent should be doc-umented, for example, via a nurse's note in a medical chart recording oral consent. In some instances, NIH considered the CRC's meeting minutes, which recorded their approval of researchers' plans to ask for consent, as an alternative to subjects' signatures on forms. As an NIH guide phrased agency leaders' position as of 1968, "Documentary evidence of informed consent may consist of a record of the decision of the committee as to the type of consent it considered acceptable." The paper record generated by human-subjects committees, in other words, provided evidence that researchers had observed subjects' right to consent—and therefore protected the institution legally—regardless of whether signed forms were used.

Today, consent is often associated with forms signed by research partici-pants that have been approved by an IRB. But informed consent was not synonymous with consent *forms* in the 1950s and 1960s. At a time when researchers had a good deal of control over crafting NIH policy, they aimed to keep their options open by building expert discretion into the rules. The Medical Board's CRC became a fixture within the Clinical Center in part because, researchers argued, an expert review body, not lawyers, had the au-thority to define evidence of consent. The work of the review board became tremendously important at NIH as part of researchers' resistance to collecting signed consent forms.

Medical Records in Science and Law

No one owned patients' medical records, and yet everyone wanted them. This combination of communalism and covetousness was evident in the gaps on the shelves of the Medical Records Department in the years after the Clinical Center opened. The charts for all patients—sick people and Normal controls—were supposed to be kept forever in a series of rooms on the ground floor of the hospital. This central holding area was a neces-sary concession among institute directors, who preferred to keep resources and services for each of their institutes separate—protected—from the other institutes. Researchers planned to share healthy patients, though, and this meant that Normals would be enrolled in studies from several different institutes during a stay.[9] Sarah, for example, was shuttled to different wards within the Clinical Center when she served on studies for the National Heart Institute, the National Institute of Arthritis and Metabolic Diseases, and the National Institute of Mental Health. In part, the collection of charts in the Medical Records Department testified to persistent crises over the Clinical Center's low occupancy rates, which hovered around 60 percent, or three hundred full beds, throughout the 1950s and 1960s. Problems in recruiting sufficient numbers of clinically interesting sick patients and Normal control patients continually plagued the hospital from the time it opened in 1953.[10]

Still, it was a challenge to lay hands on the medical records of even those people who were successfully recruited to the Clinical Center. Researchers left with the charts for other hospitals; nurses hoarded them on the wards; staffers lost them in transit.[11] There was a committee of the Medical Board dedicated to fretting over charts: why they went missing, what should be written in them, whether red ink was better than black. (Red was traditionally used for recording blood pressures; black was preferable for reproducing records for insurers, lawyers, and employers.)[12] Producing and then managing the records was a small industry. Around the time Sarah Isaac left the Clinical Center in the late 1950s, the Medical Records Department had seventy-eight employees, all of them apparently women, one-third of them professional typists. The women of the Transcription Section spent their work hours listening to the recorded voices of men who were on the hospital floors above them giving new patients their first physicals and taking their medical histories. Doctors spoke into a dictaphone words that typists transformed into a paper record. The women's fingers kept pace with the awkward medical terms that doctors made a point to enunciate, but they paused at the everyday adjectives that they did not understand—revealing the gender and class divides between scientists and their support staff. Once typists created the record, they passed it to the Medicolegal Section, which managed requests for patient information in the charts, often from insurance companies. While a patient was still in the hospital, though, doctors and nurses kept the chart on the ward, so they could write directly into it by hand. Two other sections of the Medical Records Department—Research and Statistics, and Filing—dealt with getting all of the papers from one patient into one chart and then trying to keep track of it over the years.[13] In 1964 the Clinical Center revolutionized its record-keeping practices by

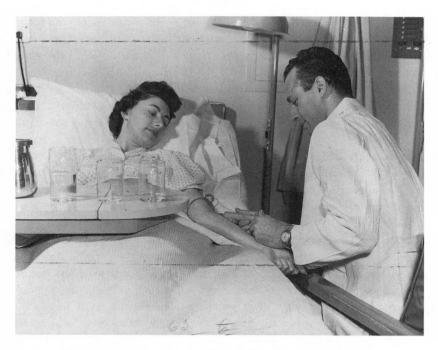

Figure 7. Mennonite Normal patient in radioisotope tracer study at the
Clinical Center, 1963. Courtesy of the Mennonite Church USA.

requiring researchers to go to the Medical Records Department to do research with charts from discharged patients, rather than letting the charts
go out to researchers. Refusing to lend out the chart was counterintuitive to
the stewards of the records, because they saw themselves as proprietors of
a library.[14] Department employees were long called "medical librarians,"
and they took seriously the spirit of lending, despite its perils at the Clinical
Center. "A hospital without records is like a clock without hands," was the
mantra of medical records librarians. "It runs but it tells us nothing."

Medical records, in other words, were objects of obsession: they were
assiduously read, stolen, amended, and fixed. NIH leaders rued the state of
their Medical Records Department, and this reveals how important patients'
charts were for two key contingents: researchers and lawyers. Their arguments over what had *not* been committed to medical charts may tell us as
much as the documents that eventually did make it into the formal record.[15]
Thus, in a nontrivial sense, most of the work at the Clinical Center was organized around record-keeping, because records produced evidence—both
scientific and legal evidence.

NIH Lawyers against Expert Discretion

Among all the things that were systematically being committed to patients' records, signed research consent forms were often, but not always, to be found.[16] This troubled Edward Rourke, the cautious and confident career lawyer at NIH. For two decades, he commuted each day to the main administrative building on the Bethesda campus, where he worked his way up the short ladder of the Office of General Counsel. He was in his early forties in 1951 when he was assigned to advise administrators on the NIH's Clinical Center Project. Rourke's new duties were stacked on top of his other NIH assignments, such as answering tax questions and explaining which foreign scientists could be employed. By 1970, nearing the end of his career, Rourke was assistant general counsel at the Department of Health, Education, and Welfare (today's Department of Health and Human Services). Advising on clinical research took up more of his workweek as the Clinical Center grew and NIH funding of clinical research boomed through the Nixon administration. Rourke spent his legal career literally in the growing shadow of the Clinical Center.

In medicine, coordinated research in hospitals was still innovative in the 1950s, and by extension, it was also unprecedented in the law. This worried Rourke. He wanted NIH to avoid being on the wrong side of one of the first lawsuits, but he also wanted to predict what evidence would seal a case in favor of researchers if a Normal control were to sue. In Rourke's opinion, the best legal safeguards were paper forms signed by sick and healthy patients, which would serve as proof that they had consented to be studied and had released NIH from liability.

Rourke's advocacy of signed forms served his professional and personal ends. As the Clinical Center's legal counsel, he felt that signed forms provided the best evidence that subjects had consented to research. Evidence of a subject's consent that originated with the researcher—whether a notation in the medical record or an intuition of consent—was less convincing than a mark by a plaintiff's own pen. As a close observer of researchers at the Clinical Center, Rourke may have thought that signed forms offered a way to curb their "pioneer" spirit, or what has more charitably been called the "can-do" attitude of Clinical Center researchers at the time.[17] Consent forms allowed lawyers vicariously to extend their will into the clinic—passing a note of caution to human subjects as they elbowed researchers aside. Lawyers never visited Sarah Isaac's hospital room, but their presence was nonetheless felt if not as strongly as Rourke would have liked, in the forms she sometimes signed.

Throughout his career, Rourke urged caution and consent forms at every turn. As early as 1952, when NIH was planning for the Clinical Center opening, Rourke attended a meeting in which the clinical directors were first writing policy for the hospital. This was a time when researchers could still write the policies that would govern them, and lawyers were guests in this process. The clinical directors had agreed, in theory, to collect signed forms for healthy patients. (The documents were called consent forms or liability release forms; the language was still flexible at the time.) Throughout the 1950s, clinicians held firm to the opinion that consent to be researched was implicit in sick people's admission to the Clinical Center and that patients' written consent was necessary only for specific procedures such as anesthesia and photography.[18] Yet even in the 1952 meeting, Rourke lobbied for broader and better-documented consent. He told clinical directors that it was "important that people doing clinical research secure overall consent for projects before the patient becomes involved." Perhaps unsurprisingly the clinical directors rejected the possibility of more expansive use of consent forms. In doing so they also marked the cleavage between employees responsible for NIH's legal defense and those charged with delivering research findings. Despite Rourke's pitch to the board, the meeting minutes described "a general feeling on the part of the research people present that routine research consent forms are not desirable." Their justification was part compassion and part self-interest: "They thought that such signed consent would interfere with the doctor-patient relationship, and also that the patient would become fearful and perhaps not cooperate as well." Rourke left defeated. "There was no consensus as to just when consent forms would be used," the meeting minutes reported, "but it was generally agreed that each case would involve individual decision and that consent forms would be used only where the project leader believed it necessary."[19] It was a triumph for the tradition of researcher discretion.

Thus, from the start of the Normals program in 1953, researchers agreed that they would get consent from healthy patients, but they did not think this necessarily meant signed forms. The recruiters or admissions staff dealt with initial liability release forms as a matter of course, just as they managed Normals' luggage, bed assignments, and general orientation to life inside the hospital. So Normals most often signed forms when they first entered the Clinical Center. Sometimes, though, forms were signed after the study was finished, which suggests that forms were thought of as having legal value to NIH more than informational value to the (presumably literate) Normals. After their first study, Normals were less likely to sign forms because they were enrolled almost spontaneously.[20] For example, when NIH administrators audited medical records of fifty-two Normal controls who lived at the Clinical Center between July 1, 1956, and May 11, 1957, they found "infrequent evidence of such informed consent." The report continued, "As a matter of fact, there is evidence that occasionally normal controls are started on new studies without notification or explanation of any kind."[21]

Sarah Isaac, for example, was first admitted to the Clinical Center in May of 1954 to start a study with James Wyngaarden (who was NIH director from 1982 to 1989). When Sarah moved into the Clinical Center, she signed a form to "apply for permission to participate in an investigation of the way in which the body handles and excretes cortisone-like substances." Provided she passed her physical, the form indicated that she agreed to live at the Clinical Center with restrictions that would vary. The second paragraph of the two-page form spelled out more details:

> I further consent freely to the intravenous administration of small volumes of solution containing the compound to be studied, and to the withdrawal of blood samples as necessary to determine the rate of metabolism of this compound, called hydrocortisone-14-C14. I also know that this substance contains a small amount of radioactivity, but that there is no radiation hazard involved, in the opinion of the Atomic Energy Commission, which has approved the experiment. The procedures, the potential benefits to humanity and science, and the inconveniences to which I may be subjected have been explained to me by Dr. James B. Wyngaarden.

The form continued onto a second page, where the fill-in-the-blank Normal (in this case Sarah) stated that she released "the Public Health Service and its personnel from liability which may result from my participation in this investigation." Sarah and two witnesses signed the form. The space for the signature of the Medical Officer was never filled.

Even if they used forms, researchers resisted standardizing consent forms for Normals. Sarah signed documents that were at once consent, permission, and liability-release forms for two studies she entered a few months later with Dr. Hiatt, who was a colleague of Dr. Wyngaarden in the National Institute of Arthritis and Metabolic Diseases. By today's standards Hiatt's consent form would be considered good, though imperfect. In one readable single-spaced page, the form described what the parathyroid gland is, what Hiatt wanted to know about it, and what the research procedures involved (a controlled diet, kidney exams, and a tricky procedure in which researchers were to give a solution intravenously at the same time that they collected Sarah's urine through a catheter). "If a subject volunteers to participate," he (yes, *he*) will be admitted to the Clinical Center and will release the Public Health Service from liability. The form also explained the compensation scheme and made mention of a study brochure that contained more details. Although the presumption of the male pronoun may sound retrograde given that Sarah signed it, the use of the conditional "if" sounds, by contrast, ahead of its time. Hiatt's form also suggests the burden on Normals to be strong readers. Rourke's ideas about legal consent relied on the presumption that Normals could learn about studies through written texts. Rourke never addressed the question of literacy, which is inherent in his advocacy of signed forms.

The differences in consent forms were more stark across institutes. In between her studies with Dr. Hiatt, Sarah was recruited for a protocol from the National Heart Institute. The "statement" she signed "certified" that she gave "full permission to the physicians of the Metabolism Section." It continued with more general terms: "I will allow blood samples to be drawn, injections of heparin, protamine, hormones, and or insulin given either intravenously or subcutaneously as the occasion might warrant." In addition to undefined physical restrictions and collections of unspecified bodily fluids, Sarah understood that "I have the right to have explained to me any experiments [to my understanding] that I think warrant an explanation."[22]

During the mid-1950s, some researchers followed Rourke's advice to collect signed forms, but they avoided standardizing the documents. This allowed researchers to retain as much discretion as they saw fit and also to defend the autonomy of their home institutes against the impositions of others. It also created a remarkable amount of work. It often happened that for each new study, a research team created a new document appropriate to the study and to the Normal control. The Clinical Center in the 1950s could be an intimate place, with few Normals and a stable cast of characters leading research. It is instructive that when Sarah moved to ward 9-West to join Dr. Savage's study as a Normal control, the form she signed had been individually typed, not set and mimeographed. The individual consent form was also one-third of the length of the others:

I, Sarah Isaac, apply for permission to participate in the study of the effects of lysergic acid diethyl amide (LSD-25) on psychic processes. I understand the drug produces a disturbance of feeling and thinking for a period of approximately six (6) hours. I further understand that the drug has been given to a number of normal people in studies similar to these and that it is safe. I therefore, agree to release the USPHS and its personnel from any liability which may result from these procedures.[23]

It was more labor-intensive to avoid standardization, unless, of course, researchers did not produce forms at all. Compared to the moment when Normals were admitted, researchers gave less priority to getting Normals to sign consent forms as the Normals passed to different institutes and as researchers cycled in and out of the Clinical Center over the years. Each institute had different routines, standards, and expectations.

In essence, researchers worked to keep consent forms within their discretion, to be tailored to fit the institute, when written consent was gathered at all. During her first year at the Clinical Center, Sarah signed five forms indicating she released NIH from liability and agreed to be enrolled in studies. She lived at the Clinical Center for an additional two and a half years, and she was on LSD studies for that period. But she never signed another NIH consent form. Sarah's state of mind, and the very meaning of the consent forms she had already signed, later came to be seen in a very different light.

Nonetheless, top NIH administrators used Rourke as their heavy, to threaten clinicians but without any real prospect of punishment for disobedience. On a bitter Thursday afternoon in January 1958, for example, Rourke was called to remind the clinical staff about the need for researchers to be careful with the Normals. Rourke made these comments a few months after a landmark decision in a medical malpractice suit, *Salgo v. Leland Stanford Jr. University Board of Trustees* (1957). Rourke was fastidious and he read around, and so he would have known of this important decision, even though there is no record of his thoughts on it. In the *Salgo* decision, the court suggested that clinicians had to tell patients not only what was going to happen in the course of the therapy the doctor recommended but also what risks and alternatives there were. Yet the *Salgo* case did not entirely apply to the work researchers did at the Clinical Center. It was a medical malpractice suit; the plaintiff had not been in a study. Moreover, as legal historians Faden and Beauchamp have written, the *Salgo* court in "a splendid burst of obscurity" wrote that physicians' disclosures to patients "should be consistent with physician *discretion*."[24] It seemed that courts might continue to defer to clinicians' expert judgment even after 1957.

In the late 1950s, U.S. courts were at least taking up questions of proper consent, even if they seemed to reentrench the authority of medical experts.

In these circumstances, it was unclear to Rourke how to proceed, given his anxiety that NIH would get sued and researchers' own resistance to formalizing consent procedures. "What am I supposed to do," Rourke asked administrators before taking the stage, "Scare them?" Apparently, yes. In the 1958 session, Rourke informed researchers that they, not NIH, would be personally liable if their research subjects sued. "You are a group of very brave people from what little I know of the law," Rourke started, with a well-played bit of self-deprecation in front of a cocksure audience:

> You are at the frontier of medicine, I assume; I know you are at the frontier of the law. For what you are doing there is no precedent in our Anglo-Saxon legal tradition that applies to the situation and I pray that you won't be the occasion for the first precedent in the courts of our country. By analogy [to] the precedents we do have it is certainly clear that to any extent that you fail to comply with either the standards such as those reported by the American Medical Association or the standards adopted by the Clinical Center you are automatically liable for any harm that arises from deliberately undertaken procedures. We are not talking about negligence or carelessness. What you are doing is deliberate.[25]

Wrapping up, he gave researchers his legal advice: "The only thing I should probably say is this—buy insurance."[26] What Rourke's warning encouraged researchers to do, however, was to make sure that they wrote policies for the Clinical Center that accommodated their research needs.

Throughout his career, Rourke saw himself as among the more "conservative" voices in legal debates about clinical research. In 1970, for example, he took Dr. Henry K. Beecher to task in the pages of the *Journal of the American Medical Association*. Rourke had been offended by Beecher and coauthor William Curran's assertion that parents should be allowed broad authority to consent for their children to be enrolled in studies. This was a bold move by Rourke. At this time, Beecher's professional and public renown was quite high. He was already a well-connected Harvard anesthesiologist in 1966 when he published an article describing twenty-two studies that he considered unethical, a piece that made him a public figure and sealed his place in the history books. In the article, Beecher's point, which is too often overlooked today, was that doctors, whom Beecher saw as generally upstanding, should be allowed to keep the authority traditionally granted them to make decisions in clinical research.[27] In Beecher's view, clinical researchers, such as himself, should not be beholden to patients' whims, much less government rules. Rourke believed that Beecher and Curran's assertion (that parents should be allowed to consent for their children with few restrictions) smacked of the sort of medical hubris that he would spend his career working against. "Mother does not always know best," Rourke chided in his response.[28] Whether discussing parents in relation to children or doctors in relation to patients, Rourke would never abide the argument that those in power acted in the best interests of their wards.

Yet in the 1960s, Beecher's confidence in the legal force of the judgment of medical experts would have seemed reasonable. Historically, courts deferred to the opinions of medical experts in cases involving care gone awry, and doctors called to the witness stand tended to agree with their colleagues as a matter of professional courtesy. Even the landmark 1957 *Salgo* case, which introduced the term *informed consent* into medical parlance, had only a symbolic effect on doctors' practices.[29] Yet Rourke was most concerned about the "untested" terrain of clinical research. The policies that any number of institutions and professional groups had put forward "represent, at best, practical judgments," Rourke felt. And, as he pointed out, practical judgments—statements that described what was already being done in hospital rooms—were not the same as law. Rourke was speaking as much to the defiant researchers next door in the Clinical Center as he was to the wider readership of the *Journal of the American Medical Association*.

NIH Researchers against Signed Forms

Researchers, however, were often reluctant to use signed forms. In contrast to lawyers, such as Rourke, researchers resisted patient-generated documentation even as the 1962 FDA Drug Amendments demanded that they start collecting signed forms for studies on "investigational new drugs." Research on these drugs accounted for a good deal of the work done at the Clinical Center, especially on Normals, but researchers reasoned that it was not productive—legally or scientifically—to collect signed forms. Their reasoning continued to reverberate in a legal atmosphere that was becoming less sympathetic to the claimed needs of researchers by the early 1960s. But bolstered by empirical evidence—evidence that was both published in medical journals and apparent in their day-to-day experiences—researchers within the Clinical Center argued that laws should not require more signed forms. At the same time, researchers at the Clinical Center expanded notions of what was legally possible by elevating the practice of group consideration as an ethical safeguard for research subjects and a legal protection for NIH.

An important premise that shaped researchers' day-to-day work in the Clinical Center was that patients were not fully rational. It was an age-old notion that sick patients were poor decision makers because they were uneducated, deluded by their disease, or just silly. This conception of the sick patient often lined up with doctors' race-, class-, and gender-based assumptions about their patients' ability to reason. And it justified doctors' spirit of paternalism toward patients at least through the 1950s. Professional organizations promoted the same logic to create and then defend a niche in the medical marketplace as it grew increasingly competitive in the twentieth century.[30]

Within this framework for thinking about sick patients, researchers argued that the problem with consent forms was that they scared patients— not through the information presented, but through the social situation that was created by asking a patient to sign a piece of paper that resembled a legal form. Of course, to members of the NIH Office of General Counsel, this was precisely the point. Signatures on forms, as Rourke regularly reminded researchers, were most likely to be considered legally effective consent in a court of law.

But patients' emotional reaction to seeing a form clouded their judgment, researchers said, even in the best of circumstances, in which a patient was smart and discerning enough to make good judgments in the first place. Recall that in 1952, the members of the Medical Board rejected Rourke's recommendation as legal adviser to the Clinical Center. He had urged them to write policy that required researchers systematically to collect signed forms for both sick and healthy patients. The Medical Board members "thought that such signed consent would interfere with the doctor-patient relationship, and also that the patient would become fearful and perhaps not cooperate as well."[31] It was this exchange that set in motion the group-consideration guidelines that left to researchers and to the Clinical Research Committee the decision whether to collect signed forms at the Clinical Center. Such decisions would be made on a case-by-case basis.

This view was evident as late as 1964, when Henry K. Beecher, the prominent Harvard researcher whom Rourke later debated on the issue of parental consent, received a letter from Irving Ladimer, who had drafted the group-consideration guidelines and the policy that created the Normals program at the Clinical Center during the 1950s. Ladimer thought Beecher might appreciate a talk he had given to drug company executives, in which he explained how consent could be documented, particularly since, in Ladimer's view, there had been "some rather naïve discussions in the literature on the question of oral and written, formal or informal, expressed or implied types." He continued, "[I] say flatly (as I have said very frequently) that consent does not become any better, does not become any more legal, because it is written." In a review of the Nuremberg Code in 1963, he had set this classic ethics code in what he thought was its proper place for Americans. Ladimer suggested "that the word 'consent' be modified with: 'either explicit or reasonably presumed.' The remainder of the first principles of the [Nuremberg Code] relating to consent contains many legal technicalities which might leave research workers open to unrealistic damage charges," Ladimer wrote. "The spirit of these precautions, however, should be preserved by language demanding a clear mutual understanding between the investigator and the subject."[32]

Signed forms would never hurt in the court of law, Ladimer felt, but they would not help scientific endeavors. A decade after the first Medical Board meetings, echoes from them reverberated in Ladimer's words as he explained, "For many purposes it may be desirable not to wave papers around and make it look like a real estate transaction or a death notice. There are other ways to get well-documented consent. Whatever is done, however, certainly must be included and incorporated in any record."[33] The documentation of appropriate consent was essential; the subject's signature was not.

For researchers at the Clinical Center, documenting consent by requesting a signature did not merit the anxiety it created, given that consent could be documented in other ways. The routine at the Clinical Center was to put in a sick patient's chart a note written by the researcher or the nurse, attesting to the consent of the patient-subject. As a transcript of a 1958 clinical staff meeting explained, standard practice was to give a sick patient "an oral explanation suitable to his comprehension of what role he is to assume, what dangers there are. There also is to be a voluntary agreement obtained from the subject as to his understanding of the project, and this shall be recorded in the medical records and also any notation in the medical records should be made as to his concern, limitations, or other such reservations which he may hold. These are the standard areas."[34] The spirit of a tacit doctor-patient relationship shaped the consent practices that clinicians used for research as well.

Clinical staff members were at the 1958 meeting to ponder the question "Where do we fit in this picture the use of normal control subjects which are a special area of this whole matter of clinical and experimental research which we do here at the clinical center."[35] Healthy patients' minds were not clouded by disease. Yet researchers pressed back against Rourke's legal advice that they collect signatures from Normals on the grounds that healthy patients were not fully rational either. To make this case, Clinical Center researchers enrolled the authority of their own scientific findings on Normals.

Experts on the "volunteer effect" concluded that Normals in fact had abnormal components of their personalities.[36] Such abnormal components did not affect their physiology, which was fortunate for the veracity of the data that researchers had gathered on Normals. However, the abnormal components of Normals' personalities did imply that the question of whether healthy patients had consented was, like sick patients, best answered by the clear-headed researcher.

One of the most useful proponents of this view for Clinical Center leaders was an acolyte of Henry K. Beecher. By 1958, Dr. Louis Lasagna had established a strong reputation of his own, particularly for his work on the placebo effect in drug studies. In the late 1950s, he had flown from Beecher's nest at Harvard and joined the faculty of medicine at Johns Hopkins University in nearby Baltimore, Maryland. Later in his career, Lasagna reversed his early views and became a vocal defender of the rights of research participants, but in the 1950s he advocated for doctors' authority.

Making just a short trip from Baltimore to Bethesda, Lasagna was one among several experts who arrived at the Clinical Center in January 1958 to address a conference on the question "How normal is the normal control?" The conference title was not an innocent question. The assembly gathered three weeks after the clinical staff meeting at which Rourke had spoken on the question of how to document consent from Normals. Regardless of the answer given to the question of Normals' normalcy, the question itself was a justification for researchers' view that they need not be more fastidious in their collection of signatures on consent forms for Normal controls. Indeed, Lasagna's research findings served to justify researchers' sense that they need not be overly concerned with Rourke's claim that courts would regard a signed form as stronger evidence of consent than a doctor's good word. Lasagna had reported in *Science* the findings of his studies of Harvard college boys, for example, which concluded that half of the subjects recruited as Normal controls showed, upon questioning, "severe psychological maladjustment." Although appalling to present-day sensibilities, Lasagna's categories of "maladjustment" reflected contemporary definitions of disease: homosexuality, alcoholism, stuttering, or the all-purpose "psychopathic personality."[37] It is also worth noting that researchers, including Lasagna, rarely considered the possibility that the drugs they were giving subjects, LSD for example, had created the psychosis they found in their Normal volunteers.

In 1958 Lasagna and his fellow conferees had a ready answer to the question "How normal is the normal control?" To the researchers gathered in the Clinical Center auditorium, the answer seemed to be "not very." The

suggestion that Normals were not fully rational, though not actually mentally ill, opened up the useful terrain into which researchers would argue the
value of the group-consideration model, especially for deciding the best way
to document consent of people they enrolled as Normal controls.

In pondering these questions in 1958, some researchers in the conference audience may have called to mind Sarah Isaac, who had packed up
her things after living years at the Clinical Center and moved out just two
months before the conference took place in the first-floor auditorium. After
her first few months at the Clinical Center, Sarah had asked for a psychiatric
evaluation. In a letter to a work-placement organization, her ward supervisor at the Clinical Center confirmed that she was unusually smart and
would make an excellent addition to a secretarial pool. Dr. Harold Greenberg explained that Sarah was seeing a therapist for mild hysteria, but that
it was nothing to be concerned about. Indeed, at the Clinical Center, Sarah
was still serving in studies as a Normal control because hysterics like Sarah
were rather commonplace. Although they were not ideal recruits, people
with everyday woes and anxieties were common enough that researchers
agreed that they were "normal" in the sense that they were in good company. Sarah served as a Normal control in studies for several institutes
while she was in therapy, including her final study as a healthy patient,
administered through the National Institute of Mental Health. In this study,
Dr. Charles Savage transferred her to psychiatric ward 9-West to serve as the
Normal control for his research into the effects of LSD on schizophrenic patients (mentioned earlier). Although Sarah had started therapy with a NIH
psychiatrist five months prior, she was still designated a Normal control to
which comparisons to sick patients would be drawn.[38]

Sarah shows that the dividing line between sick and healthy people was
unclear, even though contemporary research methods presumed that there
were obvious, categorical distinctions. Sarah's time at the Clinical Center
seemed to be drawing to a close in the spring of 1956 as Dr. Savage's research wrapped up, but Sarah did not want to leave the hospital. Although
she found the banality of her fellow Normals and the idiocy of the nurses
nearly intolerable, she was sated by the conversations with her therapist, by
bantering with the well-bred doctors, and by enjoying the generous meal
service. (She was obese. "Her need to be fed amazes me," one clinician
remarked.) Perhaps living in a hospital had affected her mind. Perhaps she
also liked the drugs by now. Regardless, in July 1956, Sarah was recatego-
rized. She had cut herself ("not in anywhere serious," doctors reported);
she started a fire in the Clinical Center (neither the first nor the last, though
Bunsen burners were a more common culprit); and she threw things at the

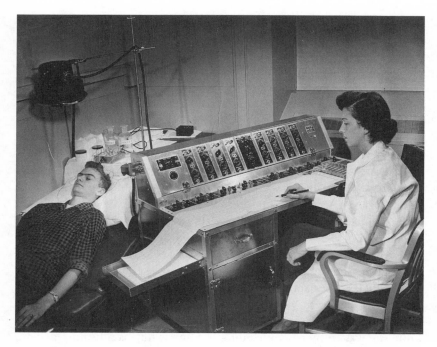

Figure 8. Mennonite Normal patient in study of LSD-25 at the Clinical Center, circa 1956. Courtesy of the Mennonite Church USA.

dinner table. To Dr. Savage, Dr. Greenberg, and Sarah's therapist, Dr. Day, such bad behavior was a possible marker that a Normal had crossed into a pathological state. And so for the next year and a half, Sarah was enrolled in various studies on sick patients. The downside was that she could no longer help to fill the short supply of Normal controls. The good news was that Sarah could stay on the same ward on which she had lived as a control for the LSD studies, by serving as a psychiatric patient in the same studies of LSD. The staff never openly questioned the veracity of their earlier data.

By 1960, NIH scientists felt they had a selection problem on their hands, which explained why Normals like Sarah might slip into the sick-patient category. The first reason they identified for Normals' pathological tendencies was that, by and large, the Normals had come primarily from Mennonite and Brethren communities during the 1950s. "The result is that there are not enough volunteers assigned to NIH," the program administrators reported, "and there is a high prevalence of psychopathology among those who come here." To NIH researchers, the church volunteers were by definition deviant: "It is also a truth that in our culture a normal young person is more likely to pursue an uninterrupted course of educational or gainful occupational self-advancement, than to dedicate a year or two of his or her life to community service." In addition, NIH administrators felt that the church sent "their most normal and effective volunteers . . . into the field to positions of independent responsibility, while 'placement problems' [were] assigned to NIH."[39] By 1965, the proportion of Normals who had to be discharged or turned into sick patients because of psychiatric problems was so uncannily high that NIH scientists began to suspect that psychotic people from all of their sending organizations were intentionally trying to get a foot in the door at the Clinical Center. Once in, they would take advantage of its excellent care. For example, in the 1964 annual report of the Normal Volunteer Patient Program, the program director noted as "Special Incidents" the discharge of three college-age Normals because of psychiatric problems. "What these actions did provide was a refocusing of attention on the policy that any volunteer, who after admission, indicates a need for psychiatric treatment will be discharged after a complete psychiatric work-up, evaluation and referral is made, rather than receive such treatment. This re-emphasis was necessary as it appeared that some students might conceivably be volunteering for services with this express thought in mind."[40]

At the Clinical Center, normalcy and consent remained a persistent puzzle with scientific and legal researchers. But they regarded these research findings not so much as a challenge to the veracity of the data they had collected. Instead, researchers regarded them as a vindication of their claim that signed consent forms would be less important in the event of a lawsuit than a researcher's judgment and testimony about whether subjects consented. In 1965 NIH organized another series of meetings to address the question of how to document consent at NIH. During one get-together, for instance, the director of clinical investigation at the National Institute of Mental Health (NIMH), Dr. Robert Cohen, reported to the group that people serving as "normal controls" had shown "irrational components in their decisions regarding their participation" in investigations. Like Lasagna's study a decade earlier, Cohen described how in one study of supposedly healthy volunteers, NIMH investigators had found that eleven out of twenty-nine Normals had shown "significant psychopathology."[41] Cohen "felt that these people should not be regarded as normal controls and [he] questioned whether a psychiatric diagnosis should be made."[42] Cohen and his colleagues used these and other studies of Normal controls to question whether even these most able-minded research subjects could give meaningful consent.

At one of the board's final meetings, psychiatrist Philippe Cardon explained the ethical implications of NIMH research experiences: "The validity of the 'informed consent' which may be obtained from patients is question-able," he explained. "It must be borne in mind," he continued, "that it is much easier to obtain the consent of a patient than of a review commit-tee."[43] It is worth noting that Cardon was among the most lax consent-form collectors at the Clinical Center. That said, Cardon's view was in keeping with the times.

In 1958, Clinical Center policy had formally changed: researchers were supposed to collect signed forms from Normals for each study at the Clinical Center. But old habits died slowly, and researchers had hardly noticed the formal policy change. Even as the congressional hearings were under way that led to the 1962 FDA Drug Amendments, the Medical Board voted *not* to require that researchers collect signed forms from Normal controls. This vote came after the Clinical Center leaders had looked over a proposed revision to the information that NIH would be providing to Normals. They con-cluded, in the words of the new director of the Normals program in 1960, "We now have a wider variety of normal controls, and the rules and regula-tions applicable in the past need modification." Dr. Clifton Himmelsbach was referring to the prisoners who would be coming to the Clinical Center in 1960 to compensate for the dearth of religious volunteers after Sarah Isaac's cohort left. Speaking for the National Heart Institute on the topic "Evidence Substantiating the Requirement That Normal Volunteers Give Signatory Consent to Participate in Research Projects in the Clinical Center," Dr. Ber-liner stated, "It was left up to the individual Institute as to whether or not the patient is required to sign such a statement. In those Institutes where this is not a requirement, the physician puts a note on the chart stating that he has explained the project to the patient."[44] The model of the sick patient, the imperative of institutes' autonomy, and the value of expert discretion permeated policies relating to the Normals program even in 1960.

The members of the Clinical Center's Medical Board agreed with Berli-ner's summary of appropriate consent practices, which did not please Him-melsbach, the new head of the Normals program. In 1960 Himmelsbach was trying to convince the Bureau of Prisons that researchers would reliably collect consent forms if the bureau agreed to send men to be studied. "The [Medical] Board's acceptance of Dr. Berliner's contrary view that signatory consent is an elective matter came as a distinct surprise and was assumed to be based on some authoritative action which had not been encountered in our review of existing regulations," Himmelsbach wrote. "In view of the explicit and implicit documentation pronouncements superseding the orig-inal elective position on gaining the signatory consent of a normal volun-teer before permitting his participation in a research project, it is requested that the Medical Board reconsider its action of October 11, 1960 on this point."[45] Even if Himmelsbach could not change what researchers actually did, he would at least change what they claimed they did.

Thus, it cannot be assumed that any formal policy changes were widely discussed or broadcast. Regarding consent documents, NIH researchers later explained that they understood new policies, to the extent that they knew of them at all, to be recommendations ("may" collect signed forms) rather than requirements ("must" collect signed forms).[46] The tinge of volunteers' irrationality was tremendously fruitful in Clinical Center leaders' efforts to stave off signed forms. Clinical Center leaders maintained that researchers' discretion was most valuable in knowing when someone had truly consented to serve in a study, especially when the patient's rationality was changing or at least open to question.

Conclusion: Forms of Consent circa 1960

During the first decade that the Clinical Center was open—from 1953 to roughly 1963—expert group review was "institutionalized" as a way of governing. To say that a practice is institutionalized means that it becomes an entrenched, routine way of doing things. Institutionalized practices gradually come to seem intuitive to their participants and come to require less justification and explanation over time. Today, researchers dislike many of the specific rules binding review boards: the rules about who serves on boards, which studies have to be reviewed, and the criteria by which research is judged. Yet this method of making decisions is itself less often questioned. Some critics of IRBs propose that group review be left to a committee within an academic department or a panel within their professional association, but an expert declarative body nonetheless.

During the Clinical Center's first decade, the discretion of group review became the legitimate, default way of making decisions about the limits of research on people. Clinicians stuck with this routine even as the congressional hearings that led to the 1962 Drug Amendments, which brought NIH under the regulatory purview of the FDA, shifted the balance toward signed forms as the legally relevant evidence of consent. Yet NIH researchers remained steady in their conviction: greater use of signed forms was ill-advised, they felt, even amid this changing legal environment of the late 1950s and early 1960s. No doubt, this was a self-serving argument for NIH scientists.

Whether it was genuine or contrived, however, they based their argument on contemporary research findings and their local experiences with

Normals at the Clinical Center, including Sarah Isaac. The Clinical Center had been home for Sarah: her community and her affections were there. But what made someone a healthy well-adjusted adult—making and valuing friendships, for example—could be cast as a pathology at the Clinical Center. Sarah, for example, wrote regularly to Dr. Greenberg, whom she called "Pop." After she moved out of his ward, Sarah still hoped he would reply to her notes, as another clinician had done. "How about you following suit?" she asked, "Not just to support my narcissism, but to encourage my flagging spirit. After all, I miss you, too, since I'm not around for your morning & evening visits. Have fun at your ward rounds this morning. I'll be thinking of you all and trusting that you'll not miss my tennis shoes on the footstool in the corner."[47] Sarah's case demonstrated that researchers had what they felt to be a legitimate claim that signed consent forms from healthy volunteers would not necessarily hold up in court because even healthy patients were thought to be mentally unreliable. What mattered more than anything else, Clinical Center leaders persisted, was the researchers' judgment as to whether Normal controls had consented.

Paradoxically, NIH researchers built scientific evidence for this legal claim using the early religious volunteers—including Sarah Isaac—who were given psychiatric diagnoses while at the Clinical Center. For her part, Sarah was discharged a schizophrenic and went on to a productive career as a secretary in Washington, D.C., only coming back to NIH to threaten a lawsuit against the agency in the 1970s during the Church Committee hearings, which exposed covert government research on LSD. Understanding researchers' serious concern over the "normalcy" of Normal controls helps to explain their reluctance to collect standardized forms as legal evidence of consent.

Although formal policy changed in the late 1950s, researchers followed the routines and practices that had been set in place when the Normals program started and the Clinical Center opened. By the late 1950s, these habits were comfortable, and the group-review technique suited their claims that experts should get to decide what counted as evidence of consent and that experts should do so on a case-by-case basis.

Clinical Center leaders eventually yielded in principle, if not in practice, to demands for signed forms. Yet the habit of creating evidence of participants' consent through standard signed forms was layered on top of the previously used method of group consideration. Clinical Center researchers expanded the importance, and the legal possibilities, of expert group review so that they could hold on to expert discretion and, in particular, discretion in deciding how to create evidence of consent.

Thus, group review was designed to allow researchers to avoid consent documents. The Medical Board's Clinical Research Committee became increasingly important at the NIH Clinical Center not because of researchers' goodwill or because of lawyers' insistence. The Clinical Research Committee was researchers' tool of choice through which they could get formal permission *not* to use signed forms. Researchers extended the importance of expert review groups during the 1950s—from minimizing risks to ensuring that subjects' rights were observed. Handing this work to NIH's Clinical Research Committee was researchers' creative adaptation of the expert-review decision-making method. Researchers did it to counteract lawyers' demands for subjects' signed forms.

SIX

Deflecting Responsibility

Changing the Locus of Lawsuits in the 1960s

Three men boarded Eastern Airlines Flight 305 out of the Washington, D.C., airport on January 6, 1961, en route to Atlanta, Georgia. Two of the men were federal prisoners recovering from an illness that they had gone to NIH not to cure but to contract. It may seem an odd order of operations: to enter a hospital in good health and to leave while recuperating.[1] But within three years, nearly one thousand prisoners would have similar experiences.[2] Throughout the 1960s, federal prisoners were flown or bussed to Bethesda to serve in malaria studies and in virus research on pneumonia, flu, the common cold, and simian virus-40.

The prisoners' smooth journey from prison to hospital ward and back again was a remarkable legal accomplishment of two government agencies. And it was enabled by the group-review system in place at the Clinical Center. The Bureau of Prisons allowed convicts to be used in studies at the Clinical Center starting in 1960, so long as NIH researchers received prior approval from the Clinical Review Committee at the Clinical Center and collected signed agreements from the prisoners.[3]

The prisoner program was also made possible by NIH administrators—most of them active or former researchers—who delicately managed political suspicions and liability threats in the early 1960s. There is no doubt that NIH was in the vanguard in developing procedures and enforcing policies that are now called human-subjects protections. When read in historical context, however, NIH's leadership on this front can be understood as an effort to deflect lawsuits away from Bethesda and toward other research sites.

NIH leaders were responding to a confluence of factors that they started to notice more acutely around 1960 and that intensified through 1964. This chapter gives witness to how NIH leaders who worked in and around the Clinical Center dealt with well-known events in the history of medical ethics, including the U.S. Food and Drug Administration's Drug Amendments in 1962 and the World Medical Association's Declaration of Helsinki in 1964. It also explains how NIH leaders understood the pressure from members of Congress regarding their use of public funding and, most alarmingly, their handling of a lawsuit concerning cancer research at the Jewish Chronic Disease Hospital in Brooklyn, New York. Pull back from the fine grain of their meetings, phone calls, and cocktails with members of Congress, and it becomes apparent that NIH science administrators had clear but complicated aims for their agency in the early 1960s: to avoid getting sued, while also protecting researchers' "scientific freedom" and continuing to be well funded with taxpayer money.

To this end, NIH director James Shannon coordinated the spread of human-subjects review committees to research institutions across the United States and abroad. In February of 1966, Surgeon General William Stewart sent a memo to research institutions throughout the country and overseas that got Public Health Service funding. In it, he informed administrators at hospitals, universities, and other research sites that they would have to set up review boards for studies on human beings if they hoped to continue getting public funding through his agency, which included NIH. By that time, legions of scientists were conducting research that NIH lawyers regarded as legally sensitive, and NIH had been implicated in a lawsuit against a cancer researcher, Dr. Chester Southam, who was funded by NIH but was not an employee. NIH would have been a casualty of its own funding success in the 1960s if it could have been sued by any research participant in a study funded through its massive Extramural Program. NIH director Shannon hoped to avoid this eventuality. As chapter 4 described, Shannon had been an early champion of the Clinical Research Committee at the Clinical Center, and as this chapter explains, he carried this model for group review to the surgeon general's desk during the mid-1960s. Thus Shannon and his colleagues exported the model of the Clinical Research Committee from Bethesda to research sites throughout the country and across the globe.

Shannon's move should not be seen simply as a reaction to NIH's political woes. Instead, it was a successful, active effort to divert liability claims away from the agency. The spread of human-subjects review was a forward-looking legal strategy on the part of NIH, rather than a reaction to current events. Viewing it in these terms makes it possible to not simply ask why ethics review emerged in the late 1960s and early 1970s; we can also understand why researchers today have *this particular* arrangement: a vast system of local review boards working at sites across the country and the world that develop local precedents, as chapter 2 explained, to suit the particular site but not to suit one another.

The Many Meanings of Prisoner Research

The legacy of the Nazis' medical war crimes reshaped American research practices in unexpected ways. The changes came twenty years after World War II ended and only after being transposed onto the context of 1960s American medicine and politics. Debates over research ethics published in both domestic and international medical journals in the early 1960s made clear that there were serious ethical concerns about research practices that had gone largely unchallenged in the United States before that time. These debates were prompted by the World Medical Association's work on international standards for medical ethics, and they showed NIH researchers that their practices were far from unassailable.

By standard accounts, modern medical ethics started with the Nuremberg Code, the 1947 document that listed ten features of ethical medical research. The Nuremberg Code was understood at the time as a shaming of Nazi doctors for their mistreatment of prisoners in the name of medicine. Although American doctors and scientists knew of the Nuremberg Code at the time, historians have established that its principles did little to change the day-to-day practice of medical research.[4] In 1964 the World Medical Association endorsed a set of recommendations for medical research practices that updated the Nuremberg Code. Contemporary researchers felt that the code was overly restrictive for researchers working with the advances of postwar medicine and, they said, too limiting for clinicians trained in democratic countries who knew right from wrong, even if they had to do unsavory things at times.

American researchers were dismayed to read a draft of the World Medical Association's recommendations written in the early 1960s, which included heavy restrictions on the use of prisoners in medical studies. The *British Medical Journal* published an early draft of the recommendations in 1962, and they were also circulated informally among Americans. Given the memories of the Holocaust in Europe, restrictions on prisoner research would seem unsurprising. And yet in the United States, prisoners fueled research on new drugs at federal penitentiaries and inside hospitals, such as the Clinical Center.[5]

At home in Bethesda, Dr. Vernon Knight read the contents of the draft recommendations and was alarmed by the restrictions on prisoner research that they proposed. Knight was clinical director of NIH's National Institute of Allergy and Infectious Disease, the hub of virus studies within the Clinical Center. As a result, Knight's institute received the largest number of prisoners at the Clinical Center, and Knight himself was a great champion of the NIH prisoner program. He published an article in 1964 in which he advocated the use of prisoners in nontherapeutic research not only because it advanced medicine but because, he argued, the experience could have "positive rehabilitative benefits" for the subjects.[6]

The NIH prisoner program started in May of 1960, and by 1966 more than 13,350 prisoners had been admitted to the Clinical Center for malaria and virus studies.[7] The prisoners who flew back to Atlanta in January of 1961 were among the first to be moved to the Clinical Center to serve as research subjects in the wards of the National Institute of Allergy and Infectious Disease. The prisoners typically stayed for either three-week or five-week terms.[8] The prisoners loved it, the program coordinator recalled. Once they got to the Clinical Center, they did not get "airline food," and it was his impression that "they had a hell of a time."[9]

It may seem ironic that research on prisoners was fueled by the new FDA drug-approval system that started in 1962, which meant that greater numbers of healthy people were needed for early-phase tests, as part of the four-phase clinical-trial system that we have today.[10] Projecting a shortfall in the number of Normals coming to the Clinical Center from historic peace churches, Dr. Clifton K. Himmelsbach had suggested that federal prisoners might fill the gap. During the 1930s, Himmelsbach had directed the prisoner research program at Leavenworth, Kansas. From there he moved to the NIH addiction research hospital in Lexington, Kentucky, where he trained under Dr. Harold Isbell, whose LSD research on prisoners most directly implicated NIH in the CIA research scandal hearings in 1977.[11] Himmelsbach studied drug withdrawal, and the Lexington hospital was a satellite research facility of the NIH Intramural Program, which housed federal prisoners addicted to drugs or alcohol. Because of his extensive experience with prisoner programs in Lexington and Leavenworth, Himmelsbach was brought into the Clinical Center in 1959 to set up a prisoner program on the main campus. By the 1950s, Himmelsbach had a strong network of contacts within the Bureau of Prisons. He and Bureau of Prisons director James V. Bennett were close friends, for example. Himmelsbach plugged Vernon Knight into his network, and he selected the first federal prisoners from a penitentiary in Pennsylvania. The Bureau of Prisons agreed to the arrangement in which NIH moved prisoners to the Clinical Center. They were "locked up, under our supervision, but there would be a federal prison guard there all the

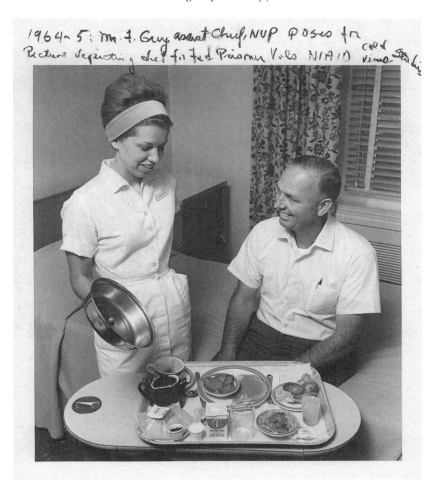

Figure 9. Federal prisoners lived at the NIH Clinical Center for three-to-five-week rotations as Normal controls in the virus research for the National Institute of Allergy and Infectious Disease. The writing on this photo reads, "1964–5: Mr. F Grey, Assistant Chief, NVP [Normal Volunteer Program] poses for picture depicting diet for fed[eral] prisoner vol[unteer]s NIAID cold virus studies." Courtesy of the National Institutes of Health, Office of Patient Recruitment and Public Liaison, Building 61.

while," Himmelsbach recalled in 1994. "Actually the experience was good, I don't think a single one got away. They just enjoyed the hell out of it because they were away from prison at the NIH where the food was better and everything was better."[12]

Memories can deceive. A few prisoners did slip away from the Clinical Center, but it is unclear how far they got or where they hoped to go. Delbert

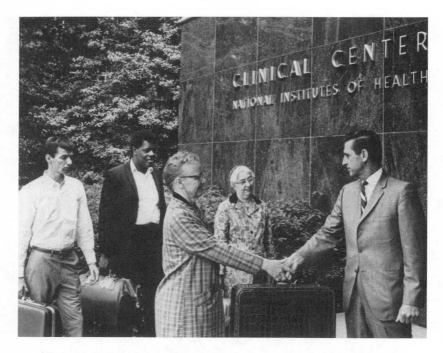

Figure 10. Delbert Nye, two Normal control volunteers recruited for osteoporosis studies, and their porters, circa 1966. Courtesy of the Mennonite Church USA.

Nye, who was the head of the Normal Volunteer Patient Program in the 1960s and a master of euphemism, reported that prisoners were involved in several "misadventures" during the early 1960s. Just before Christmas 1964, for example, two federal prisoners took "unauthorized leave" from the Clinical Center. The following year, Nye reported, "Security measures were recently strengthened on the 11 East Nursing Unit [a prisoner unit], and custodial force furnished by the National Training School for Boys is now headed by a Lieutenant, Correctional Services." These improvements may have been precipitated by a "special incident" that he did not describe in detail but that resulted in a prisoner's being sent back to the penitentiary. The same year, Nye reported, a Normal control from the Brethren Volunteer Service "inadvertently" gave a prisoner the keys to a church bus. "The volunteer in question alleged he did not know the patient was a federal prisoner."[13] At least in his written account, Nye did not ponder the fact that pacifist church volunteers seemed always to have a knack for nonviolent resistance to authority.

NIH researchers knew that prisoner research was unsavory to some on-lookers, and yet prisoners were an essential resource for their studies at the Clinical Center.[14] During the mid-1960s, NIH avoided mention of the Clinical Center's prisoner program in public venues, even as convicts arrived in Bethesda from more than a dozen penitentiaries and served as many days in the Clinical Center as all other Normal control patients combined (around nine thousand days annually).[15] To give a sense of the scale of the prisoner program, in the 1964–65 fiscal year prisoners served 8,974 man-days at the Clinical Center, and they served 9,868 man-days the following fiscal year.[16] In other words, there were on average twenty-six prisoners living in the Clinical Center on any given day between 1964 to 1966; around 8 percent of the beds that were full had prisoners in them. Just as interesting as the numbers, though, is the method NIH administrators used to keep track of the prisoners in-house. Note the metric of man-days, rather than men, and the time frame of the fiscal year rather than the calendar year. The administrators thought in terms of expenses—time is money, as they say—and in terms of necessary resources for scientists' research at the Clinical Center.

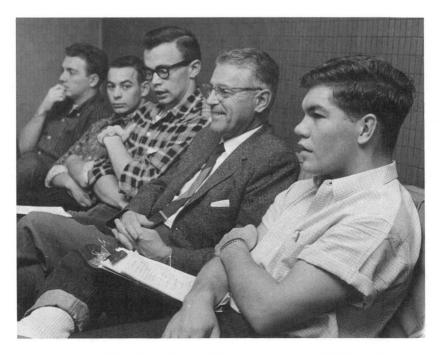

Figure 11. Dr. Clifton Himmelsbach with Normal patients at the NIH Clinical Center.
Courtesy of the Mennonite Church USA.

It was a banner year for prisoner research in 1964. The NIH Clinical Center admitted its one-thousandth prisoner, and the World Medical Association published its final recommendations for medical research, known as the Declaration of Helsinki. In the end the declaration was as notable for the activities it allowed—namely, prisoner research—as for the practices it restricted. Leaders of the World Medical Association in Europe had planned to curb research on prisoners, as described earlier. American researchers disliked this restriction in the early draft, and, importantly, American medical organizations were major funders of the association. As historian Susan Lederer has documented, American medical leaders worked to remove restrictions on prisoner research from the World Medical Association's recommendations before the document went up for approval in 1964. For the time being, then, Vernon Knight and his colleagues working in the prisoner wards at the Clinical Center could rest easy. NIH's research enterprise continued to expand through the 1960s as it tapped more Normal controls and as congressional appropriations grew. Nonetheless, the work of NIH researchers on the main campus in Bethesda did not sit comfortably with the moral sensibilities to which NIH was now being exposed.

Public Money and NIH Liability

Dr. Jack Masur was the first director of the NIH Clinical Center, overseeing the prisoner program and much more at the facility during his long tenure. He was appointed director in 1952, before the Clinical Center even opened, and held the post until March 8, 1969, the day he died of a heart attack. Masur was remembered for his "endearing belligerence"—the rare NIH administrator who used capital letters and exclamation points in his writing.[17] Masur is beloved at the Clinical Center today: his portrait hangs by the entrance to the main auditorium, which is named in his honor. In the early 1950s, James Shannon appeared already to respect Masur. As a newly appointed NIH director, Shannon enlisted Masur when he was looking for a new head of the Clinical Center with an aggressive leadership style.[18] Their careers at NIH overlapped for almost two decades, Masur as the head of the Clinical Center and Shannon as director of the entire NIH agency.

During his tenure as Clinical Center director, Masur rarely assigned required reading for the Medical Board, the group of senior researchers who set NIH policy for clinical research in Bethesda. But in February of 1964, Masur urged the Medical Board to read an article from the latest issue of *Science*, "Human Experimentation: Cancer Studies at Sloan-Kettering Stir Public Debate on Medical Ethics."[19] He brought copies. It was that important.

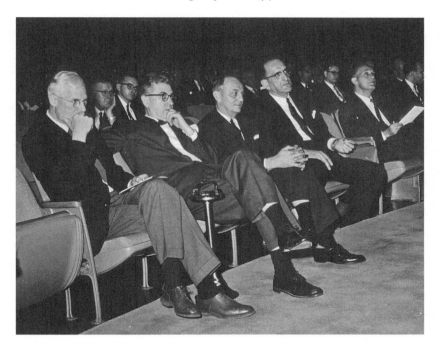

Figure 12. The three men in the middle of this photo, Dr. James A. Shannon, Dr. Luther Terry, and Dr. Jack Masur, spoke often and knew one another well. Here they listen to a lecture in the Clinical Center auditorium, which is called the Masur auditorium today. They are flanked by Dr. Richard L. Masland (*left*) and Dr. Seymour Kety (*right*). Photo by Robert S. Pumphrey. Courtesy of the National Library of Medicine.

In 1964 members of a new profession, science journalism, reported on a case in which two physicians had injected twenty-two patients at New York's Jewish Chronic Disease Hospital with cancer cells without first getting their consent.[20] Within a community that included many Holocaust survivors, it was particularly upsetting to learn that clinical researchers had injected the patients as part of a study supported in part through NIH's National Cancer Institute. Because of this funding connection to NIH, the attorneys for the defendant hospital demanded that the Public Health Service (the parent organization of NIH) indemnify the hospital for the damages that it might have to pay to at least one elderly and arthritic plaintiff, Mr. Fink.[21] Lawyers for the plaintiffs had argued that the key researcher funded through NIH, Chester Southam, had not followed the procedures outlined in the Clinical Center's group-consideration guidelines. NIH lawyers successfully explained that researchers funded through the Extramural Program were not bound by the Clinical Center's local policy.[22] This time NIH did not have to pay up, but the legal attention to the Clinical Center's group-review practices prompted worry and defensiveness on the main campus.

By 1964, funding had created two major problems for NIH. First, members of Congress charged that NIH was not using public funding responsibly and questioned in general terms whether researchers' judgment should be trusted. This did not bode well for deference to researchers' authority on ethical and legal matters. Second, Senator Jacob Javits (R-NY) learned about the Jewish Chronic Disease Hospital scandal in his state and pressed NIH to adopt standard practices for collecting written consent from research participants, much as he had urged the Food and Drug Administration a few years earlier. When the FDA was in disarray from congressional hearings during the early 1960s, NIH leaders had spent the time trying to safeguard their agency against external regulation and rigid consent documentation (see chapter 5). With mounting pressure from Congress and lawsuits looming, NIH director James Shannon deflected legal responsibility—and thus financial risk—for NIH-sponsored research outward to the institutions that it funded in 1966. The Clinical Center's Clinical Research Committee became the solution to another problem for NIH leaders, this time by providing a model for expert review outside of Bethesda.

Public Funding in the 1960s

NIH's National Cancer Institute funded the study that prompted the research scandal at the Jewish Chronic Disease Hospital in New York. The vast increase in funding to NIH starting in 1956 was significant in part because of the health research it enabled. This funding increase also served to consolidate Shannon's power, to boost the number of American investigators beholden to federal research policies, and to heighten congressional scrutiny of and influence over NIH.[23] Although Shannon was the driving force behind what even he regarded as the "unorthodox . . . and quite unprecedented" funding boom for NIH, he was aided by health research enthusiasts in Congress, many of whom were well positioned on appropriations committees and were pursued tenaciously by an emerging health research lobby.[24] In particular, Shannon was a friend and drinking companion of Representative John Fogarty (D-RI), chair of the House appropriations subcommittee that ushered NIH funding through the House. Shannon characterized their friendship by saying he knew Fogarty "more on a personal than a technical basis."[25] Shannon had a less intimate but nonetheless fruitful relationship with Lister Hill (D-AL), who was Fogarty's counterpart in the Senate (and whose father was Dr. Luther Terry's namesake). By 1960,

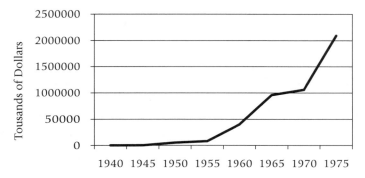

Figure 13. NIH appropriations, 1940–1975. *Source*: NIH Almanac, www.nih.gov/about/almanac/historical/index.htm. *Note*: Data are in constant dollars.

Shannon had established a direct line past the surgeon general of the Public Health Service (PHS) and the secretary of the Department of Health, Education, and Welfare (HEW) to the House and the Senate, such that he "seemed to answer to nobody but Congress."[26]

Although Shannon and his congressional allies assured lavish funding for NIH, by the early 1960s some fiscal conservatives worried that Congress was, in the words of Representative Melvin Laird (R-WI) "force feeding" the institutes, particularly their extramural investigators, more money than they could responsibly use.[27] NIH supporters argued that Shannon was running a tight ship, and they used as evidence the fact that in some years NIH had returned to the U.S. Treasury money that it could not soundly spend. They also claimed that NIH sponsored only meritorious extramural research based on the recommendations of its celebrated study sections. Congressional conservatives countered that NIH was a piratical operation, with an administration that was unable to keep abreast of budget responsibilities and that acquiesced too easily to investigators' demands that the federal government stand clear of the research it funded.[28] During congressional hearings in 1962 on the issue of NIH spending, Shannon in particular appeared to rely on the rhetoric of investigators' scientific freedom at the great expense, literally, of the federal government.[29] In one especially infelicitous—and revealingly raw—moment, Shannon alienated otherwise sympathetic legislators by dismissing the suggestion that NIH investigators needed to be held accountable for their spending.[30] What really mattered, Shannon testified, was selecting "good men and good ideas," which NIH was doing through its study sections. Other considerations, like investigators' money management, Shannon said, were "essentially trivial."[31] After having issued a "mildly worded" and more or less forgettable report in 1961 that called for more efficient spending practices, Congress's Fountain Committee in 1962 responded to Shannon's inaction and perceived arrogance during the hearings.[32] Representative L. H. Fountain (D-NC) found enough support in Congress to push through new requirements that required grantees to document their spending more precisely. The new requirements prompted NIH's first extramural *Grants Policy Manual*, which was part of an effort intended, according to Shannon, "to clarify the moral obligations of the scientist as a trustee of public funds."[33] The new requirements also stirred an impressive amount of vitriol among investigators receiving word of the new oversight.[34]

In response to the Fountain Committee's report, President John Kennedy, and later President Lyndon Johnson, assembled the independent Wooldridge Committee, which in its own 1965 report generally praised NIH budget management but called for changes in the decision-making system that continued to reverberate within the NIH. The Wooldridge Committee encouraged NIH to decentralize many responsibilities then cloistered in Bethesda to the local universities and hospitals receiving extramural grants and to solicit advice on matters of public interest from "scientists and laymen [who] will provide an essential assurance to Congress, to the scientific community, and to the public at large that the great powers of the Government are not being unwisely or arbitrarily employed."[35]

For observers, the results of the hearing had implications beyond the question of NIH spending habits. It demonstrated that for those outside of the health research world, it was "hard to accept NIH's view that the ethical standards of the scientific community are a sufficient safeguard" against any number of misjudgments.[36]

NIH Safeguards: The Law-Medicine Research Institute and the Livingston Committee

Thus, Shannon was considering the advantages of relocating the administrative and moral responsibilities of research to the home institutions of his extramural investigators. From 1960 through 1963, NIH funded work by the newly created Law-Medicine Research Institute at Boston University to study whether hospitals and research universities had proper procedures in place to protect research participants.[37] The study was led by Irving Ladimer, a longtime friend of the Clinical Center and a former NIH planning department employee (see chapter 4). One Law-Medicine survey sponsored by

NIH found that only a small number of the institutions had committees of scientists in place as of 1960.[38] When Ladimer asked journal editors about ethics policies they used, most deferred to professional societies in medicine "or referred to the general expectation that clinical investigators would do nothing to harm the patient, create unnecessary risks, or infringe upon the patients' rights." Ladimer reported, "Most editors decided on the basis of `common sense,' treating each instance individually." He summed up what he found in the early 1960s: "Although the editors were aware of ethical problems inherent in clinical research, their lack of specific standards or policies indicated that they have not considered these problems to be frequent or significant enough to demand their formal concern."[39]

In 1964 Shannon also asked NIH staff member Dr. Robert Livingston to chair a group on the treatment of research volunteers, which was to report to him on the "professional . . . patterns of practice in this delicate area."[40] He wanted the Livingston Committee, as it was called, to suggest changes that NIH could make to manage its complicity with investigators in their use of humans as objects of study. Among their four recommendations, Livingston and his colleagues encouraged Shannon to gather more information about how procedures for protecting people were actually carried out in universities and hospitals. They also encouraged Shannon to commission a "professional group" to formulate principles "relating to the moral and ethical aspects of clinical investigations."[41] Several months later, Shannon disavowed the view that NIH should draw up principles for the treatment of human subjects, remarking that "the Public Health Service is not searching for another code."[42]

Shannon did not lose sight of the fact that NIH was funded with public money, which made the agency vulnerable to lawsuits from people at the sites where studies took place, whether they were elderly cancer patients or federal prisoners. The funding arrangement also made NIH open to criticism from the legislators who appropriated the money in the first place.

Senator Javits and the Threat of Written Consent

In the summer of 1965, lawmakers approached the Public Health Service with explicit concern about protecting the rights of research subjects. Leading the charge was Senator Jacob Javits, who started his campaign at the top of the PHS organizational chart with Surgeon General Luther Terry. This was an important episode for the Clinical Center because it brought the Clinical Center's group-review procedure into the mainstream medical press, revealing that many NIH administrators, lawyers, and investigators sharply disagreed on the issue of how decisions regarding the use of humans in clinical research should be made.

Javits was already well known, even infamous, within the health research community by 1965. He had frustrated many medical scientists several years earlier by inserting, controversially, strict consent requirements into the 1962 FDA Drug Amendments for researchers testing unlicensed drugs on people.[43] In the summer of 1965, Javits cast his eye toward the PHS (which at this time did *not* include the FDA). After Javits became concerned about PHS practices because of the lawsuit against the Jewish Chronic Disease Hospital in his home state of New York, he asked Terry, "Does the experience of your Department suggest the desirability of legislation extending the 1962 [Drug] Act consent provisions to all Federally regulated or financed experimentation and research?" Terry's answer was a rather indignant "no."[44]

Terry held firm to the view, reminiscent of the opinions of investigators serving on his Medical Board when it wrote the 1953 group-consideration guidelines, that the country was best served by leaving investigators unfettered by government restrictions. He told Javits, "We should avoid to the utmost utilizing the grant-in-aid relationship as a mechanism for exerting Federal control and direction." Again echoing the sentiments of his old Medical Board, Terry informed Javits that the best protection for research participants was the investigator's good character and thus his sound judgment, which only his scientific peers were equipped to gauge through an evaluation of his professional talents: "The prime consideration in respect to safeguarding of patients involved in federally supported clinical research is the integrity, sense of responsibility, and stature of the investigators and institutions to which Federal support is provided. The process of review of such activities for scientific merit by scientific peers which is provided for through the Public Health Service framework of study sections and review panels helps to assure such qualifications," Terry wrote, acknowledging the primacy of peer judgment. "Therefore, I have confidence," he continued, "that the clinical research and experimentation carried out through this grants-in-aid support is characterized by recognition of the ethical and moral obligations of the patient-physician relationship which is the foundation of relationships in medicine and medical science." For intramural research, meanwhile, there was "clear procedure for the obtaining of informed consent," Terry told Javits. Here Terry was referring to the 1953 group-consideration guidelines that were still in place. Terry did not explain that these guidelines were flexible on the issue of how to document the fact that consent had been obtained, explained in chapter 5.[45] To further ease Javits's concerns, Terry assured him that the National Advisory Health Council, which was his advisory group as surgeon general, planned to take up the issue of human-research protections in the coming months.

In 1965 Javits also forwarded to Clinical Center director Jack Masur a news article on the Jewish Chronic Disease Hospital and a letter of concern from a constituent. Masur responded to Javits with words very similar to Terry's. Although Masur acknowledged the "grave ethical, legal, professional, and moral problems involved in these increasingly complex situations," he nonetheless maintained, "Fundamentally we must depend upon the integrity, conscience, and the conscientiousness of the physician in charge of the patient."[46]

Shortly thereafter, Alanson Willcox, the general counsel of the Public Health Service (and Edward Rourke's supervisor), read the correspondence between Javits and Terry from the summer of 1965. Willcox was "troubled" by Terry's response. The surgeon general seemed to be "indicat[ing] that there are no problems at NIH."[47] Willcox, by contrast, was "certain that NIH is beset by the same uncertainties" that Terry had claimed investigators could manage without federal oversight. The uncertainties, for Willcox, included "the real nature of informed consent, what constitutes clear evidence of consent, what degree of hazard can an individual consent to," and the question overarching all of these, "whose judgment is necessary and sufficient as to what these limits are." Willcox discussed the Javits-Terry exchange with Rourke and learned that Rourke also felt that Terry had "take[n] on too much," particularly with the "glowing assurances of integrity and ethics of grantees and our confidence in them. Too much has and can happen."[48]

Rourke's skepticism about the good judgment of investigators had been reinforced by his personal involvement in *Fink v. Jewish Chronic Disease Hospital*.[49] Rourke most clearly articulated his policy ideals for NIH through this case. He felt that investigators could not be trusted to obtain legally binding consent from the people they studied, no matter how closely the process was legislated. The best he could do, then, was to remove the Public Health Service from responsibility for its grantees.

Rourke suggested this option to Surgeon General Terry in September 1965 when he recommended that PHS require contracts—what he called "assurances"—with investigators in which they would certify that they would treat their research subjects appropriately. How investigators and their institutions defined appropriate treatment was less of a concern than simply making the issue someone else's responsibility. Rourke's goal was "to make expressly clear that this PHS does not supervise or control the conduct of research it supports by grants." In this spirit, he enticed Terry, assurances would "help define what responsibilities you have undertaken and, perhaps of greater value, what responsibilities you have not undertaken."[50]

Terry was perhaps the closest thing Rourke had to a nemesis. Terry had been an advocate of unchecked scientific freedom since his early days at the Clinical Center. Meanwhile, Rourke continued to argue, as he had in 1953, that investigators should be required to ask people's permission to use them in studies and to obtain a signed consent form in nearly all circumstances. He felt that this would both protect PHS against lawsuits and force investigators to observe what he felt were people's legal rights: in his words, "the competent patient's or subject's free right to control the use of his person whether the purpose be diagnostic, therapeutic or research." In contrast to investigators, Rourke embraced subjects' seeming irrationality: "Only the individual with all his ignorance, superstitions and foibles, can make the important choice [to be researched] and, being fully informed as possible, he is free to make it for particular reasons or for no reasons at all." The implications, for Rourke, were that researchers should not be allowed to make consent determinations for other people, that researchers were incapable of recognizing their hubris regarding consent, and that if people were not allowed to consent for themselves, public protest would ensue. Rourke remarked, "Although the judgment of a scientist's peers may be important to him, it is hardly the judgment he or the scientific community need be most concerned with. The judgments that will in the long run have the significant impact on clinical research will be those of the courts, Congressmen, trustees and other `lay' representatives of the public. What I feel is overdue is recognition by the medical scientist that he will not ultimately make the rules that will govern his work in this area."[51] It is easy to imagine that Rourke included himself among the lay representatives to whom he referred.

Deflecting Legal Liability

As NIH director, James Shannon shared the faith in researchers' good judgment held by Terry, Masur, and many top scientists at PHS. But Shannon also recognized the value in ceding some ground to lawmakers. In this spirit, Shannon developed a new human-subjects policy, this one for extramural researchers, during the autumn of 1965, to help manage growing congressional concern over informed consent. Although it was neither ideal for investigators nor exactly what lawmakers had in mind, Shannon crafted a policy that was nonetheless acceptable to both groups. Instead of accepting the informed-consent requirements promoted by Javits and his supporters, Shannon adopted a compromise position, in which he imposed the NIH tradition of group consideration on the sprawling extramural program. This policy ushered in research oversight for most American universities and hospitals and, at the same time, limited federal intrusion into scientists' research practices by neutralizing calls for rigid consent requirements.

Through the autumn and winter of 1965, Shannon coordinated a campaign to force universities and hospitals to promise that they would be responsible for protecting sick and healthy people enrolled in studies at their institutions. As Terry had promised Javits, the National Advisory Health Council discussed the matter at its late-September meeting.[52] Terry attended the meeting—he was presumably the one being advised—even though he had already announced his resignation and was turning over his duties three days later. The official story is that Terry was pulled away from the PHS by a prestigious offer from the University of Pennsylvania Medical School, where he remained until the end of his career, though it is tempting to read more into Terry's resignation at a moment of polarized debate with members of Congress in which he held a politically unpopular view. One of Terry's subordinates, William Stewart, was selected to replace him as surgeon general. Stewart was quickly confirmed, despite his own surprise that he had been appointed and the general sense that he was an unusually junior choice for the post. Stewart's rank may have made him particularly amenable to the policy suggestions of the more experienced Shannon.

At the autumn meetings of the National Advisory Health Council, Shannon presented on the use of human subjects in research, arguing that moral judgment "cannot be the exclusive responsibility of the investigator." Still, Shannon did not take an overly imaginative view of who should be involved in science decision making in the public interest. In his presentation, Shannon carefully avoided the insinuation that investigators had acted irresponsibly with research subjects or the public in the past. Taking a page from the Livingston Report, he framed the present need for an explicit policy as the product of new research methods, which had brought new practices and new objects of study into the investigator's purview. Shannon argued that past research had been based on "observation" but that this method was "being replaced by manipulation," or experimentation. Describing the randomized controlled trial, Shannon explained that the new method required "not only the diseased individual but normal individuals," who are "used as guides to the understanding of abnormal states." Involving people in research *because* they were healthy created a new relationship that stood outside of most codes of ethics and traditional invocations of the sacred doctor-patient relationship. The consequence of changing research methods,

Shannon asserted, was that any PHS-sponsored investigation "should be discussed with a peer group," that is, peers of the investigator, "for a basis of sound judgment." Shannon did not mention an alternative: namely, that investigators should always get and document participants' informed consent before proceeding. At the end of the Advisory Council discussion, Shannon offered that "NIH would continue with quiet explorations of the subject," which meant that he would develop a human-subjects protection policy.[53] Shannon consulted specifically with Rourke, redrafted with small revisions the resolution that he had previously proposed to the Advisory Council, and got the council's final approval of the resolution on December 3, 1965.[54]

The beginning of human-research review in American universities and hospitals is commonly traced to 1966, the year during which Surgeon General Stewart issued three memos that announced and then detailed the review procedures required of institutions employing PHS grantees. In his first memo on February 8, 1966, Stewart quoted the recent resolution by the National Advisory Health Council—now his advisory group—and informed major universities, hospitals, and professional associations that to receive money from the Public Health Service, they would have to "provide prior review of the judgment of the principal investigator or program director by a committee of his institutional associates." It was up to this committee to review risks, benefits, and protection of patients' rights, as well as to assess "the appropriateness of the methods used to secure informed consent." Stewart made no mention of how consent should be documented. It is important to note that Stewart did not circulate guiding principles but instead told grantees, "The wisdom and sound professional judgment of you and your staff will determine what constitutes the rights and welfare of human subjects in research, what constitutes informed consent, and what constitutes the risks and potential medical benefits of a particular investigation."[55] The standard material of ethics codes—risks, benefits, and consent—were not defined but were to be, according to Stewart, whatever the local committee deemed appropriate.

Stewart imagined that without standard principles to guide review committees' evaluations, their good judgments could be ensured through their membership. Thus, he took special care to "define more explicitly" who could rightfully be considered an investigator's "associate." For Stewart, an associate needed to be a university or hospital employee or consultant who was "acquainted with the investigator under review" but who, despite this personal familiarity with an investigator, was "sufficiently mature and competent to make the necessary assessment" and possibly able to represent "different disciplines or interests that do not overlap those of the investigator under review."[56] Stewart was ventriloquizing Shannon's view that a range of disciplinary perspectives should be represented on review committees because of concerns that conflicts of interest would be rampant in insular groups.

In 1966 the NIH Extramural Program was extensive, and this new human-subjects review policy affected a large number of investigators, touched most American research institutions, and quickly became the talk of the science community. In response to investigators' reactions, most of which ranged from alarm to confusion, Stewart circulated a double-edged follow-up on July 1, 1966, the second of his three policy memos. It further extended the reach of the policy to cover nearly all PHS grants, rather than just the research and training grants he had originally targeted, but it also routinized the procedure for "group review." Whereas each investigator had previously been given the opportunity—or burden—to create a fresh human-subjects review committee for each project, Stewart now advised creating one permanent committee at each institution to assess all investigators. This was meant to allow "agreements between each grantee institution and the Public Health Service which will obviate the necessity for providing detailed assurance with each application."[57]

Stewart's third memo on human-subjects research, in December 1966, was a reply to investigators doing nonmedical research. He particularly addressed psychologists who worried that the new policy would limit the use of deception. He clarified at this time that the new requirements for extramural research did indeed apply to social and behavioral scientists.[58]

NIH leaders had taken Javits's threat seriously because he had successfully forced consent requirements on FDA-regulated investigators in 1962 and because NIH was operating at a perilous time—at a moment, for example, when international medical leaders registered their displeasure with American prisoner research and when patients sought to hold NIH liable for the actions of the researchers the agency funded. However, although NIH leaders were increasingly pressed to impose rigid consent requirements on their own vast cadre of extramural investigators, NIH director James Shannon and his administrative colleagues instead imposed decentralized, local ethics review committees on universities and hospitals. Shannon pushed for procedures, not principles. Although "more sophisticated" principles could be written than those available in 1965, Shannon thought that investigators did not need "another formulation."[59] The key point of similarity between the Clinical Center's Clinical Research Committee and the models that the surgeon general extended to research institutions nationwide was that local review committees were charged with adapting the meaning of informed consent and its appropriate documentation on a flexible, case-by-case basis.

Conclusion: An Ethics for Other Places

At the NIH Clinical Center during the 1950s and early 1960s, the Clinical Research Committee provided a technique for solving legal problems, as much as a method for making moral decisions. Clinical Center leaders aspired to allow scientists to explore new areas of clinical research and also wanted to maintain a positive reputation for the Clinical Center among members of Congress, journalists, and American citizens. This was especially trying in the early 1960s as news broke of abusive research on Jewish patients funded by NIH's National Cancer Institute. At the same time, NIH leaders angled to prevent outside regulation and to safeguard biomedical research as Congress forced the Food and Drug Administration to tighten its regulations on human-subjects research and as the World Medical Association announced international standards of research ethics. Within their building itself, Clinical Center leaders aimed, as always, to protect the resources of their individual institutes—whether floor space, man hours, or Bunsen burners—while finding a way to share the resources that they could not individually possess, such as medical charts, laundry service, and Normal control subjects. The group-consideration guidelines that Clinical Center leaders created in the early 1950s and institutionalized into the 1960s served all of these purposes.

In the early 1960s, however, the Clinical Center's old guard was beset with new problems. By now, many of them had moved even further up the ranks. President Kennedy nominated Luther Terry, the former Medical Board director, as surgeon general in 1961. James Shannon retained his directorship of NIH and secured unprecedented amounts of funding for the agency—in effect building a powerful research agency underneath his own feet. However, the amount of public money flowing toward NIH opened the agency's accounting practices to unpleasant scrutiny from fiscal conservatives in Congress. The bounty of public funding that arrived every budget season starting in 1958 meant that NIH had been able to sponsor studies on humans at hundreds of research sites across the United States and abroad through its Extramural Program. Yet, research subjects were holding NIH responsible for the exploits of researchers who were supported by these funds and thus brought to the fore questions of NIH accountability and research consent. The money NIH was giving out now put the agency on the receiving end of expensive lawsuits, as well as unseemly intrigue.

By the end of the 1960s, most American research universities, hospitals, and institutes had group-review procedures in place because the surgeon general had made committee review a condition of funding starting in 1966. Soon, group review was required not only by the NIH but also by the FDA. Political scientist Daniel Carpenter aptly describes the expansion of ethics review boards in the 1960s as the creation of "satellite regulators" by the National Institutes of Health in its 1966 policy and by the Food and Drug Administration through its own regulations three years later.[60] Paradoxically, FDA's 1962 Drug Amendments prompted much of the research on prisoners at the Clinical Center that was so contentious as the World Medical Association wrote new standards for research ethics.[61]

Today's institutional review boards are direct descendants of the Clinical Research Committee that met inside NIH's Clinical Center starting in the 1950s. In 1971 the secretary of the Department of Health Education and Welfare (later renamed Health and Human Services) adopted the surgeon general's 1966 policy for the entire department, not only the Public Health Service. This created even more inertia for the group-review decision-making method, which ultimately was mandated by the federal human-subjects regulations passed in the 1974 National Research Act. Indeed, NIH administrators submitted group review as a suggested model while the research bill was being put into place between 1973 and 1974. And it is no coincidence that the federal Office for Protection from Research Risks—the office that was created to enforce federal human-subjects regulations at local sites—was in Building 31 on the NIH campus, across the street and down-hill a few paces from the NIH Clinical Center.[62]

Charles McCarthy, who led the Office for Protection from Research Risks in its early years, recalled the importance of NIH's Clinical Research Committee. "The policy [of group consideration] required oversight of research involving normal volunteers by peers in the Clinical Center," McCarthy explained. "The policy that Shannon recommended to the [National Advisory Health Council] in 1965 borrowed and expanded the Clinical Center policy to all research subjects involved in both intramural and extramural research." Then, under time pressure to come up with regulations when the Tuskegee Syphilis Study story broke in 1972, policymakers adopted the DHEW rules wholesale. "Although the new regulations were little different in content from the DHEW [policy]," McCarthy wrote, "they enjoyed the force of law."[63]

Expert groups were invented at NIH in the early 1950s, entrenched through the next decade, and spread onward and outward beginning in 1966. The success of this model was fueled in part by the increasing scale and complexity of human-subjects research in the 1950s and 1960s. Even more significant, though, were the new civic concerns and research funding structures that prompted NIH leaders to extend the group-review model from the Clinical Center to other research sites and into the future.

The Making of Ethical Research

A Way of Deciding

There was not much good news to be had in June of 1966. American bombers were striking Vietnam, a civil rights activist was murdered in Mississippi, and medical researchers across the country had been running questionable experiments on people. This last piece of bad news came from the pen of renowned Harvard anesthesiologist Dr. Henry K. Beecher, and it rocked the world of research.

But this was a world that was ready to be rocked. In 1959 Beecher had published a similar article enumerating research abuses, and he had given lectures on the topic in recent years.[1] At this earlier time, Beecher's words had a considerably smaller effect both on practitioners and on public opinion. What a difference a few years can make. In 1966 Beecher published a very similar article in the *New England Journal of Medicine*, and this is the piece for which he is remembered and celebrated.[2] This curious fact says a great deal about the differences between his audiences in 1959 and 1966. The earlier readers glanced past Beecher's news, but the later readers seized on his cases and made them scandals.

Thus, Beecher is memorialized in the history of medical ethics because of the way his words were read and understood in the political and social context of 1966. By that time, the civil rights movement had sensitized Americans to recognize how people with little power could be exploited by traditional authority figures, including doctors.[3] In the academy, philosophers and theologians were carving out a niche for a new profession called bioethics. The federal government under the Johnson administration was taking steps to open more decisions to public scrutiny. In the present-day literature in bioethics, Beecher's article offers a convenient reference point to mark a groundswell of American activism about human-subjects protections, which developed in the mid-1960s. Beecher's article surely contributed to this upsurge. But it is just as fair to say that American moral and medical sensibilities in the late 1960s lifted the article to prominence.

Four months before the article appeared in medical school mailboxes, Beecher had learned that he was bound by a new federal policy. The policy required that an expert body at Harvard give prior approval to his proposed research on human subjects.[4] In February of 1966, the surgeon general notified hospitals, universities, and other research institutions that they had to set up human-subjects review boards if they wanted to receive—or continue receiving—federal funding for research. This was the culmination of a longer process that fundamentally altered how research decisions were made.

Over the previous two decades, NIH researchers, lawyers, and administrators had created, institutionalized, and extended a procedure designed to protect research subjects from harm and exploitation. At NIH they were motivated as much by liability concerns for the agency as by their moral vision of human rights. The aim of this book is not to diminish the value of their work, but to draw attention to the distinctive features of the group-review model they created and to point out how it might have been different.

In the early 1950s, researchers at NIH were keen to cultivate a positive image for the fledgling agency, whose funding was entirely dependent on congressional appropriations. NIH researchers thus aimed to make efficient and careful use of a resource that was essential but scarce: humans who could be enrolled in studies. They created a routine that they hoped would ensure that not only sick patients, but most importantly "healthy patients"—their term for civilians, conscripts, and prisoners who legally could be studied at NIH—did not get hurt in experiments, for example by being used simultaneously in too many studies or enrolled in studies researchers regarded as especially risky. They called this decision-making technique group consideration. It involved prior review of a study by a few men on the Clinical Center's Medical Board: research directors, leaders of individual institutes, and their colleagues.

At the time, it was an unusual way of making a decision about how a scientist should act, because choices were not left to the individual researcher, following his professional code of ethics. The group-review model did, however, preserve the great virtue of profession-based ethics: deference to expert discretion. The group-review model also suited the Clinical Center and its location within the federal government, because it became attached to activities within the walls of the research hospital, creating what I call "an ethics of place."

Researchers at the Clinical Center attributed more virtues to the decision-making procedure later in the 1950s and early 1960s when NIH was particularly strained to create documentary evidence of consent from sick and healthy patients. Group consideration assured Clinical Center leaders that they had legally relevant proof that research subjects had consented in the most appropriate manner—which the committee got to define. In some circumstances, they reasoned, the most appropriate form of consent would be spoken words, in other circumstances it would be signatures on paper, and in rare instances consent would be evident in subjects' actions, such as allowing themselves to be admitted to the Clinical Center. In light of contemporary questions about the meaning and the public repercussions of collecting signed forms from people, researchers opted for a procedure that privileged expert discretion. The present-day sense that a signed form represents a participant's authentic consent was layered on top of the review-board model. Today human-subjects regulations still give IRB members a good deal of discretion in deciding what kind of evidence researchers need to collect to prove that their participants truly consented, even if IRBs rarely use this legal flexibility.

Eventually, NIH did draw lawsuits in the 1960s, not from healthy patients in the Clinical Center as lawyers had feared, but from subjects in studies funded through the NIH Extramural Program, which did not take place on the Bethesda campus and were not conducted by NIH employees. Most provocative for NIH leaders and the Office of General Counsel was the lawsuit prompted by researchers at the Jewish Chronic Disease Hospital, which was funded through NIH and had unmistakable resonances with Holocaust research for recent immigrants and Americans who were confronting, belatedly, the extent of the Nazi war crimes twenty years earlier. For the time being, Congress continued to fund NIH generously, and agency leaders were able to maintain the pool of healthy human subjects with the help of churches, universities, civic organizations, and federal prisons across the country. But the NIH clinical research program was a precarious success. In this political setting, Director James Shannon, who by this point had become legendary for his administrative cunning, hatched another savvy legal move to protect his agency. To deflect legal liability away from the agency itself and toward the institutions NIH funded, Shannon forced research institutions across the United States to reproduce the expert-review model that he had helped create for the Clinical Center before it opened in 1953. Shannon shuttled this group-review policy to the National Advisory Health Council, which pushed it on to the surgeon general, who announced in 1966 that henceforth all research institutions would need to create local expert-review bodies in order to get federal funding. This was the announcement that Henry Beecher had received at the Harvard Medical School months before his celebrated article was published.[5]

Rethinking Bioethics and Its History

The classics in the field of bioethics suggest that this new profession, while in its infancy in the late 1960s and early 1970s, imposed research regulations on biomedicine.[6] By that account, bioethics consolidated around theologians, scholars, and scientists working as moral regulators of medical research, which had become troublingly detached from Americans' collective values. One of the great early triumphs of bioethicists, by this account, was their imposition of research regulations in 1974 through the National Research Act.

From the perspective of a bioethicist, it makes sense that expert review would seem to be an outcome of the work of the founders of the modern profession. All professions have origin stories that serve to build a collective identity and a sense of solidarity among group members. Shared stories are retold, for example, in textbooks to train new members or during ceremonies marking entry into the professional world, and they allow initiates to imagine the professional community to which they now belong.

It is more historically accurate, however, to say that the invention of bioethics as a profession and the invention of expert review are two parallel stories with one common cause: medical researchers' concerns over their legal liability in clinical studies and clinical care. The establishment of expert review, on the one hand, and bioethics as a seemingly independent moral regulator, on the other, both helped researchers to manage a legal crisis that threatened their share of the federal budget and the reputation of medical researchers.[7]

Revisionist scholars have shown that medical schools and research institutions underwrote and promoted departments and training programs in bioethics. Leaders in the field of medicine, in other words, nurtured and sustained bioethics programs in an effort to rebuild the public's waning trust in practitioners. They aimed—successfully, in the main—to create a sympathetic overseer that accepted the basic premises of medical research and practice, including the postwar assumption that research on healthy citizens was essential. It is no coincidence that the physical and institutional locations of most university bioethics programs today are not in seminaries or humanities programs, but inside medical schools. Far from being medical outsiders, bioethicists were consummate insiders, this recent literature has shown. Medicine and bioethics were not inherently antagonistic; they were mutually sustaining.[8]

What, then, explains the creation of group review, if not the handiwork of bioethics? I have argued that this method of research regulation, enacted in law in 1974 on the heels of the Tuskegee Syphilis Study exposé, was an extension of a model created at NIH in the 1950s. Before the 1974 law was passed, some members of Congress had proposed an alternative to the local-review model, which was to institute one centralized federal board. NIH leaders worked behind the scenes with their allies in Congress to kill this option, in large part because it seemed likely that NIH would become the regulator, making the agency legally responsible for the actions of myriad researchers at the thousands of universities, hospitals, and research institutions it funded in the United States and abroad. The role of legal lightning rod was precisely the position that NIH leaders aimed to avoid. For agency leaders, simply turning the NIH policy of 1966 into the new federal law of 1974 was the best solution to a bad situation at the time, when Congress insisted on some form of regulation. The legacy of this brilliant political one-upmanship remains with us today.

Creating a Common Sense

When new laws are put in place, is it because they articulate a prevailing sensibility? Or do new laws reflect the interests of political elites who use their positions of power to reshape the legal terrain? It depends on the circumstances, of course, and many acts of political force are for the better, as in the case of President Johnson's strong-arm executive orders to advance civil rights in the 1960s. Over generations, people's sensibilities can start to conform to laws that were forced into place. Again, civil rights is a good example: Johnson used his presidential power to force states to observe voting rights and desegregation rules. It was a contentious move at the time and prompted public uprisings. Today, it would be unthinkable to protest voter equality or school desegregation, now that the ideals of minority rights have become entrenched.

Regarding research ethics, the prevailing wisdom among scientists and scholars today is that federal regulation for research review needs improvement, and federal officials would appear to agree—even though they are making improvements at the speed of bureaucracy. Undergirding the criticisms of the current system, however, is the basic assumption that some form of expert review is important and necessary, both to double-check the sound judgment of young researchers or fringe scientists and to legitimate the research enterprise. Part 2 of this book has documented how federal scientists (acting in their capacity as administrators and policy writers) created and extended review procedures during the 1950s and 1960s because the procedure relied on expert discretion rather than on the latest views of politicians or members of the public. Group review was compatible with NIH leaders' aspirations for postwar science. By quietly creating a new method for governing research, scientists were able to conduct studies in ways that may have been useful but were contrary to common sensibilities at the time. Researchers have started to take for granted that expert review is not just one way among many, but is *the* way, to make research ethical. Perhaps this explains the urgency in critics' demands that the government improve the current review system: it seems unthinkable to replace it with a different system altogether.

Viewing our present-day circumstances as a product of the past shows how our current arrangement could be different. One could imagine a research code that individuals would apply themselves, or a single centralized federal review body instead of thousands of local boards. Placing the past alongside the present also shows how the conversations we have (and cannot have) today with our doctors, colleagues, and potential research participants are products of a method of making decisions developed in the 1950s and 1960s.

Today research is made ethical by a network of what I have called declarative bodies. IRBs can define studies as acceptable through the say-so of knowledge experts—the physicians, academics, lawyers, clergy, and others who interpret the law at the bidding of the government. These knowledge experts make regulatory decisions to meet bureaucratic needs that are specific and temporary, for example by evaluating grant proposals, reviewing clinical-trial data, and revising school curricula. Although knowledge experts do the work of applying state regulations for a few hours per week or per month, they rarely think of themselves as bureaucrats.

Bureaucracy today, as a result, might best be thought of as a discursive setting in which speakers adopt the language and logic appropriate to the task at hand, rather than as a physical location. The aim of part 1 of this book was to explore how knowledge experts struggle in the discursive setting of the IRB meeting to create the impression that they have used fairly the discretion they have to exercise in applying abstract rules to concrete cases. For knowledge experts, working in groups helps to create the sense that their decisions are fair because they are beyond the choice of an individual. It is a remarkable social achievement that people gathered around a conference table can create the impression of having one voice. In service of this end, formal documents come in handy. Documents such as letters, meeting minutes, and memos help to leave the impression that a decision was made by one social actor, such as "the IRB." This in turn liberates IRB members to advocate more incendiary actions than they would otherwise have suggested, since individual members cannot be held accountable. Thus, documents are tools that give power to declarative bodies and authority to their say-so. At the same time, the work of creating the image of one social actor erases the accountability of the individual experts who are in fact responsible for the decision outcome.

Creating unified decisions is a remarkable accomplishment precisely because different knowledge experts have legitimate claims to valuable insights on different topics. I argue that knowledge experts manage this circumstance by warranting their opinions and thereby working to persuade other members that their views are worth endorsing as the decision of the entire group. In the IRB meetings that I observed, members were particularly swayed by opinions that colleagues warranted with their firsthand experiences, both personal and professional. In my interviews with board members, however, they only hinted at the persuasive power of firsthand knowledge derived from their personal lives (as parents, friends, neighbors, and teachers) or professional lives (as researchers who had seen-it-with-their-own-eyes). In practice, the ways in which the board members I observed reached their decisions differed markedly from the socially appropriate answers that other IRB members have tended to report in surveys or to remember when recounting discussions.

In addition to particular warrants, the group history that board members shared also shaped their decisions. Since IRBs are attached to institutional settings and empowered to make discretionary choices, the boards are prone to site-specific prejudices as a matter of organizational design. In their efforts to make consistent decisions and to work more speedily, for example, IRBs tended to treat some of their previous decisions as exemplars, specifically those that were contentious but eventually were settled firmly and by consensus. I call these exemplar decisions local precedents, because members tended to use them as model decisions that they reapplied in future cases. Local precedents help to explain the sense among researchers that the review system operates unevenly (some say unfairly). Boards seem inevitably to reach different decisions about similar studies at the thousands of research sites in the United States and abroad because each board has a unique history of cases, members, and struggles.

A decision-making model that stabilized in the 1950s and 1960s may seem out of step with present times. Researchers today often work at many sites, collaborate with colleagues across institutions, or do work that cannot be limited to one physical setting. In addition, the obligations that individuals, communities, companies, and governments have to one another extend across the political boundaries that organize national-level research regulation. I have tried to show that our current method for reaching decisions is historically contingent and to point out its best and worst features, which are often one and the same, depending on one's role within the review system.

NIH's postwar strategy for research governance shapes the way that clinical and social science is regulated today, because groups of individuals—IRB members—are required to apply abstract laws to concrete research plans. Their moves from abstract law to specific case are always acts of interpretation. Call it discretion, creativity, or a good hunch, IRB members use latitude each time they apply a regulation, which might make the range of possible decisions seem nearly limitless. Yet the *ways* in which IRB members go about making decisions is systematic because of the constraints of their social configuration: they offer warrants, apply precedents, scrutinize documents, and produce records of their own. Thus, what undergirds the individual choices of group members is a more regular decision-making process. Inside IRB meetings, that process tends to encourage research that fits with existing personal and local sensibilities about the appropriate limits of research on people. Those limits are worth reconsidering over time.

ACKNOWLEDGMENTS

Many people helped and trusted me during the course of my research. Most of them I cannot thank by name. For this reason, I am all the more grateful to the IRB members who allowed me to interview them and to observe and record their meetings without prospect of reward or credit. Several board chairs and administrators at the sites I studied also gave me food, work space, and good leads during my trips. Thank you for demonstrating such generosity.

I have had the good fortune of great colleagues and mentors at four institutions: Princeton University, Northwestern University, the National Institutes of Health, and Wesleyan University. Robert Wuthnow, Liz Lunbeck, Michèle Lamont, and Mario Small shaped this project in its early incarnation. The faculty and graduate students in Princeton's Department of Sociology and Program in History of Science created a wonderful place to learn. I thank Angela Creager for all-around support and good ideas, and I owe my subtitle to wordsmith Michael Gordin.

At Northwestern University, Ken Alder was an ideal mentor. The kindness of graduate students and faculty members in the Program in Science in Human Culture and in the Department of Sociology helped me become genuinely comfortable exchanging ideas for the first time. I am especially grateful to Sokheing Au, Chas Camic, Wendy Espeland, Gary Fine, Carol Heimer, and Art Stinchcombe. I received great advice on early drafts of this book from Alan Czaplicki, Michaela DeSoucey, Kerry Dobranski, Corey Fields, Steve Hoffman, Terry McDonnell, and Berit Vannebo. Thank you for the feedback and much more.

This manuscript started to take shape through a Stetten Fellowship at the National Institutes of Health's Office of NIH History. Dr. Robert Martensen, the director of the office and my mentor, continues to be a source of advice and encouragement. Robert has been a model of scholarly integrity that I have been lucky to witness. I thank David Cantor, deputy director of the Office, for his feedback and good humor. Finally, I thank the staff and fellows at the Office of NIH History: Eric Boyle, Brian Casey, Hank Grasso, Barbara Harkins, Chin Jou, Sharon Ku, Dan Lednicer, Michele Lyons, Sharon Mathis, Todd Olzewski, Sejal Patel, and Doogab Yi.

One of the many benefits of the Stetten Fellowship was that I learned of informal archives on the NIH campus and got to spend time with the stewards of NIH history. I am grateful to Mandy Jawara and Denora Dominguez at the Office for Patient Recruitment and Public Liaison; Trish Coffey, Michelle Hendery, James Schermerhorn, and the staff of the Medical Records Department; Charlotte Holden and Suzanne Pursley-Crotteau at the Office for Human Subjects Research; Dr. Alison Wichman; Dr. Alan Schechter; Richard Mandel at the Office of the Director; Valerie Bohen at the Office of General Counsel; and Ezekiel Emanuel and Christine Grady at the Clinical Center Department of Bioethics. NIH is a treasure trove of formal archives as well, both at the Office of NIH History and at the National Library of Medicine, where Stephen Greenberg, Michael North, Mike Sappel, and Crystal Smith helped me immensely.

I owe special thanks to Dr. John Gallin, the director of the NIH Clinical Center, for supporting my Stetten Fellowship through the Clinical Center. Finally, I am indebted to Dr. Richard Wyatt, deputy director of the Office for Intramural Research at NIH, for his encouragement and advice, especially on chapter 4.

My new colleagues at Wesleyan University have shaped my thinking already. Joe Rouse gave me much-needed advice on the history of bioethics. Jonathan Cutler helped me think through earlier versions of chapters 5 and 6. Robyn Autry workshopped chapter 1 with me. Gary Shaw gave feedback on several chapters and lent books, ideas, and courage. Many excellent students at Wesleyan have helped my writing and thinking, as well. I give special thanks to Stephanie Aracena, Erin Kelly, Alexandra Wang, and Jisan Zaman, all of whom read and commented on the entire manuscript. I owe special thanks to Lauren Feld and again to Erin Kelly to for their tireless and trustworthy research assistance. I remain indebted to Eliana Theodorou for her skill, candor, and dedication as a reader and researcher.

Several audiences improved the arguments I present in the book. I thank Matt Wisnioski and colleagues at Virginia Tech; Erika Milam and colleagues at the University of Maryland; Susan Lindee and colleagues at the University of Pennsylvania; Ben Hurlbut and members of the STS Circle at Harvard University; Adam Hedgecoe and colleagues at Cesagen, and my friends at the Public Affairs Center at Wesleyan. I am also grateful for the kindness and intelligence of Karen Darling at the University of Chicago Press, who saw me through this project. Lois Crum and Gary Morris helped me immensely through their editing.

In addition, a few important mentors and like-minded researchers have helped me along the way. I am especially grateful to Alison Winter, Jill Morawski, Robert Dingwall, Sarah Igo, Jamie Cohen-Cole, Ben Hurlbut, John Evans, Jill Fisher, Sarah Tracy, Susan Silbey, Sydney Halpern, and Rena Lederman. Friends have sustained me, too: Sarah Dry, Kathryn Lachman, Tara McCormick, Tania Munz, Kate Preskenis, Erin Sines, Anna Zajacova, and Bethany Gooch (who is not only my dear friend but my sister, too). My friend Debbie Becher deserves special mention because she gave generous comments on drafts of several chapters and gave me the term *declarative bodies*. Finally, I thank Rick, Val, Zac, and Heather for their enthusiasm.

This research was sponsored by grants through the Charlotte W. Newcombe Foundation and the National Science Foundation and a through a Wesleyan University Project Grant. I also benefited from the help of excellent librarians and archivists outside of NIH. I thank Janice Goldblum at the National Academy of Sciences; Suzanne Junod and John Swann at the FDA history office; Richard Peuser and the staff at the National Archives and Research Administration; Scott Poclosky, Jack Eckert, and colleagues at the Countway Library of Medicine; Lori Wise at the Mennonite Central Committee; Ken Shaffer, Dan McFadden, and Denise at the Brethren Historic Library; Anne Yoder and Wendy Chmielewski at the Swarthmore College archives; Rich Preheim, Denis Stolez, Natasha, and Andrea at the Mennonite Historic Archive; and Suzy Taraba, Val Gillispie, Kendall Hobbes, and many other library staff members at Wesleyan University.

My greatest thanks go to my loving family members. Alistair Sponsel's ideas and advice have informed every page of this book. Over the years that I have been working on this project, Alistair has also given me a priceless gift: he has allowed me sometimes to pretend that I am fearless. I thank my lucky stars for Beth, Marcus, Sam, Ava, and my grandmothers, Violet Wright and Joan Morris. Finally, I dedicate this book to my parents, Gary and Vi Morris, with love beyond measure.

Ethnographic Methods

My analysis is based on observations of meetings and interviews with members of three university IRBs between March 2004 and October 2005 and on twenty interviews that I conducted with IRB chairs at major research universities across the United States. For the IRB chair interviews, I drew a random sample of 20 percent of the 151 universities ($N = 30$) categorized as "doctoral/ research universities—extensive" according to the *Carnegie Classification of Higher Education*, 2000 edition, www.carnegiefoundation.org/Classification. I had a 67 percent response rate, yielding 20 interviews. The nationwide interviews provided a broad view of the common issues and modes of operation of IRBs in the United States. I also used the contacts that I made through these interviews to select the boards that I subsequently observed.

The first board, which I observed for five months, was one of several IRBs within a medical school at a university that had additional boards for non-medical research. That IRB, which I call Adams Medical Board, met twice per month for three to four hours; during those meetings I took field notes by hand. I also interviewed ten of the eleven regular members of the board, plus one nonvoting administrator. The other two IRBs that I observed were at universities without medical schools (although investigators nonetheless conducted vaccine trails, physiology studies, and other medical research), and each was the only board at its institution. At the board that I call Greenly IRB, members gave me permission to audio-record their monthly meetings for one year. I supplemented these recordings with handwritten field notes and interviews with eleven of the fourteen board members. At the other pan-university board, Sander State IRB, members gave me permission to audio-record their monthly meetings after my fifth month with the board. Thus, I recorded meetings, which averaged just under two hours, for the remainder of the year (seven months) and continued taking handwritten field notes. I also interviewed the twelve regular members of the board over the course of the year.

I transcribed the audio recordings of these nineteen meetings using the transcription conventions described below. Then I analyzed the transcriptions using the qualitative coding software Atlas.ti. The note citations of the meeting transcripts in the text follow this style: board name, month: string location in Atlas.ti. The audio-recorded transcripts list the board name for Greenly and Sander as "SG" and "NG," respectively. I chose these board names for analyzing and citing transcripts before I chose the pseudonyms, which is why the long and short names differ. For example, SG, Aug: 333. The IRBs that I observed are referred to in note citations as "SG" (Greenly State) and "NG" (Sander State). Interviews from the IRB sites are cited in the notes using "D" and "B," respectively.

Transcription Conventions

[overlapping talk; start of first speaker's words

]   overlapping talk; end of second speaker's words

[ ]   the word or phrase inside closed brackets has been altered from the actual word or phrase that a speaker used, to maintain confidentiality

/   interruption between people or one speaker's self-interruption or false start

—   trailing-off sentence

=   contiguous words; no interruption, but also no space in the conversation

( )   inaudible phrase or word that has been paraphrased based on field notes

h   one second of laughter

IRBs observed.

	Greenly IRB	Sander IRB	Adams Medical
Duration of observations	12 months	12 months	5 months
Meeting(s) per month	1	1	2
New full-board protocols in period[a]	40	20	60
IRB members			
Community members	2	2	2
Faculty and administration	12	11	9

Note: The meetings at Greenly IRB were recorded for 12 months and at Sander State IRB for 7 months. Field notes were taken during all of the board meetings.

[a]The number of full-board protocols reviewed is rounded to protect the institutions. During the meetings, all of the boards also discussed expedited protocols, study amendments, and continuing reviews.

ABBREVIATIONS

AAA	American Anthropological Association
ACHRE	Advisory Committee for Human Radiation Experiments
CC	Clinical Center
CRC	Clinical Research Committee of the National Institutes of Health's Clinical Center in Bethesda, MD
HEW	U.S. Department of Health, Education and Welfare (Renamed the Department of Health and Human Services in 1979)
FDA	U.S. Food and Drug Administration
IRB	Institutional Review Board
MCA	Mennonite Church USA Archives
NARAII	National Archives and Research Administration II, College Park, MD
NAS	National Academy of Sciences Archive
NIH	U.S. National Institutes of Health
NVPP	Normal Volunteer Patient Program, Clinical Center, NIH
PHS	U.S. Public Health Service

NOTES

INTRODUCTION

1. Willard Maginnis to Clifton Himmelsbach, January 6, 1961, "Report," PRPL, NIH.
2. Inmates were relocated from prisons to the NIH campus during the 1960s, but NIH also sponsored research on prisoners before and after this period through the extramural program. For the authoritative study of prisoner research in the United States, which includes an excellent bibliography of contemporary accounts, see Harkness, *Research behind Bars.* For examples of studies on viruses approved for prisoner experiments at the Clinical Center, see the meeting minutes of the Medical Board, Clinical Center, NIH, starting in 1960. For example, the minutes of meetings on February 9 and September 6, 1960, document approval of prisoner studies at the Clinical Center on respiratory syncytial virus; primary atypical pneumonia virus (Eaton virus), and simian virus. These minutes also include interesting discussions of a local problem with prisoner research: sick children at the Clinical Center were picking up the viruses which prisoners had been infected with for study. The minutes of September 6, 1960, record that Clinical Center director Jack Masur, who was delighted by the prisoner program, in light of a projected shortage of healthy research subjects from other organizations, suggested that J. Edward Rall, the chairman of the Clinical Center's Medical Board, write a thank-you note to Harold Janney, the medical director of the Bureau of Prisons, "expressing the Board's appreciation for his cooperation in the recruitment of normal volunteers from the Federal prison system for certain of our research studies." The chairman of the board requested that the executive secretary draft such a letter to Dr. Janney. A draft of the letter, which assures Janney that all studies are approved by a review committee, is attached to the meeting minutes from September 1960. Accession 0791, Med Board, NLM, NIH. Duplications of most of the meeting minutes of the Medical Board are also at NARAII in RG 443, Records of the NIH Clinical Center (entries 41–43 in finding aid A1), boxes 1 and 2. Details of the prisoner program are in the Clinical Research Volunteer Program's history files, located in the upstairs filing cabinet in Building 61 on the NIH campus. I am grateful to the staff of that office for giving me access to its informal archive of reports, letters, and photographs.

   For examples of published, peer-reviewed research findings based on prisoner studies at the Clinical Center, see Alford et al., "Human Responses"; Kasel et al.,

"Infection with Equine Influenza Virus"; Wyatt et al., "Acute Infectious Nonbacterial Gastroenteritis."

3.   Lederer. "Research without Borders."

4.   Sociologist Jenny Reardon has articulated this point very well in *Race to the Finish*, 162: "Phenomena, such as human genetic diversity, cannot emerge as objects of study independent of moral and social decisions about who we are what we want to know. In other words, objects simply cannot sustain critical scientific scrutiny if there are no stable moral and social orders to 'prop' them up. Consequently, technoscientific objects do not precede research projects; rather they are crafted in the very process of constructing the normative regimes needed to accommodate them. They are not preexisting neutral entities, but rather human achievements that encode particular epistemological and normative commitments."

5.   IRBs are empowered under the Code of Federal Regulation, 45 CFR 46. Statistics are from the Office for Human Research Protections (OHRP), personal communication, January 26, 2010. There were 3,771 domestic IRBs with active research registered with OHRP as of that date. On for-profit IRBs, see Emanuel, Lemmens, and Elliot, "Research Ethics Boards as For-Profit Enterprises."

6.   See Weber, *Economy and Society*, chap. 3, part 19, on the limits of direct democracy and the need for an administrative state to sustain the image of objective rule of law when many people are involved. Weber argued that democratic administrative states are contradictory because large organizations (including the administrative agencies in governments) are organized hierarchically and only people from particular social classes and status groups can serve in roles at the top of the hierarchy, which makes the organization and governance of democracies themselves undemocratic. Objectivity, in the case of administrative law, describes decisions that are "rational," that is to say, made by following rules. Again, this specific conception of objectivity (as formal rationality) comes from Weber's theory of bureaucracy. On the contradictions of the ideals between democracy and the rule by experts, see Turner, "The Problem with Experts."

7.   Lipsky, *Street-Level Bureaucracy*. Lipsky originally coined the term to critique abuses of power in police work, in particular. Lipsky's 2010 edition updates and expands his thinking on illegitimate uses of bureaucratic discretion.

8.   For examples of "commensuration," see Carson, *Measure of Merit*; Espeland, *Struggle for Water*; Espeland and Sauder, "Rankings and Reactivity"; Espeland and Stevens, "Commensuration as a Social Process"; Espeland and Vannebo, "Accountability, Quantification, and Law"; Evans, "Growth of Principlism"; Gusterson, "The Auditors." Also see Strathern, "New Accountabilities," in her foundational edited volume on audit cultures, *Audit Cultures: Anthropological Studies in Accountability, Ethics, and the Academy*. These scholars implicitly and explicitly build on Porter's argument in *Trust in Numbers* that science is not inherently quantitative but that sciences have valorized quantification because numbers are useful to governments. Quantification is a way of translating bodily perceptions—sights, sounds, touches, tastes—into existences outside of the scientist's body, which makes it appear that there is no personal influence on the process (see, e.g., Alder, *Lie Detectors*). (In addition, numbers make it convenient to govern people who are far away, because numbers can be collected and moved from the place where they are created, a useful feature for empire-building. See Latour, *Science in Action*, esp. chap. 6.) The important point here is that science and democracy have an affinity because a lack of personal influence is valued in both settings; thus science and democracy reinforce the rhetoric of objectivity in

each other. (The classic text is Shapin and Schaffer, *Leviathan and the Air Pump*. See especially chapter 7 on how the political values in Restoration England influenced what was seen as proof of natural facts. For more a recent theoretical framework for understanding the relationship between science and democracy, see Jasanoff, "Ordering Knowledge, Ordering Society," in her *States of Knowledge*). The high regard for impersonal outcomes in science and government came about around the turn of the nineteenth century. Daston and Galison, *Objectivity*. These authors also argue that conceptions of objectivity expanded and made room for scientists' judgment during the twentieth century—which may suggest that scientists have also been given more discretion in making decisions on behalf of the state.

9.   Scientists often experience a tension in their claim of a desire for autonomy from the state and their desire for political relevance and material rewards that come from being funded by the government, either as internal researchers (for example at the Food and Drug Administration, the Environmental Protection Agency, and the Department of Health and Human Services) or as outside grantees. See Carpenter, *Reputation and Power*; Freidson, "Professional Control"; Jasanoff, *Fifth Branch*; Kevles *Baltimore Case*; Mukerji, *Fragile Power*; and Stryker, "Rules, Resources, and Legitimacy Processes," 852.

10. Katznelson, "Knowledge about What," 28; Levitan and Taggart, *Promise of Greatness*; MacKenzie and Weisbrot, "The Federal Colossus."

11. On the politics of representation in expert groups, see Brown, "Fairly Balanced"; Hurlbut, "Experiments in Democracy"; and Jasanoff, "Ordering Knowledge, Ordering Society." For additional examples of groups of knowledge experts in practice, see Bosk and De Vries, "Bureaucracies of Mass Deception"; Bosk and Frader, "Institutional Ethics Committees"; Brenneis, "Discourse and Discipline"; Evans, *Playing God?*; Jasanoff, *Designs on Nature*; Keating and Cambrosio, "Who's Minding the Data?"; Lamont, *How Professors Think*; Mallard, Lamont, and Guetzkow, "Fairness as Appropriateness"; Waddell, "Reasonableness versus Rationality." Other declarative groups to which these findings may usefully extend are college admissions committees (Stevens, *Creating a Class*), religious counsels (Wilde, *Vatican II*), appeals courts (e.g., Polletta, *Freedom Is an Endless Meeting*), and film review committees (Grieveson, *Policing Cinema*).

12. Brenneis coined this perceptive term in a study of decision making within funding panels and reflection on "bureaucratic selves." Brenneis, "Discourse and Discipline."

13. With a nod to Max Weber, Kennedy explains that "formalized substantive rationality" has expanded in the United States since 1970. See Kennedy, "Logically Formal Legal Rationality."

14. Cambrosio and colleagues call this "regulatory objectivity," drawing from their innovative insider study of data safety and monitoring boards: Cambrosio et al., "Regulatory Objectivity." As legal scholar Duncan Kennedy explains, the defining feature of modern law for Weber is that law is impersonal ("enacted law" as opposed to rule by tradition, values, or emotions). There are two components of legal formal rationality (that is to say, following what rules say rather than what people say). People first write rules ("rulemaking") and then apply those rules ("lawfinding"). In practice, however, these two activities are connected, because applying rules involves giving abstract rules meaning, which in turn creates rules. Kennedy points out that the important trick in modern law, as Weber rightly notes, is to make the application of law seem impersonal, and thus fair. Rationality has the appeal of not being

subjective; decisions are beyond the judgment of any one person, and so they fit well with democracies and the imperative to rule by law. However, scholars have taken rational, object rule to mean, and to be operationalized in the state as, rule by numbers. Kennedy argues that it is a mistake to understand democratic, nonsubjective rule in such a limited way. There are more permutations. Numbers reign in some cases—namely those in which decisions are publicly exposed, with individual accountability. However, rationality also means expert groups: decisions are also outside any one person or individual subjectivity.

15. See especially Koch, *Administrative Law and Practice*, 47. The theory is that groups of experts will work as a "decisionmaking community" whose ultimate decisions can be respected and considered legitimate because they include "different personalities, agendas, value systems, types of expertise and experiences, etc . . . often by design" (8–9). It is worth noting that the past four decades have seen an increase in laws that encourage greater government transparency and accountability, including the Freedom of Information Act (1966), the Federal Advisory Committee Act (1972), and the Government in the Sunshine Act (1976). These laws might best be seen, however, as a mark of how extensive government restrictiveness and secrecy can be, rather than as remedies to the restrictiveness. One consequence of de facto limits on accessing government information is that it is difficult to study the powerful groups that make public decisions.

16. I am drawing on J. L. Austin's work on performativity, *How to Do Things with Words*. Austin's classic example is actually "I now pronounce you man and wife." I have taken the liberty of updating. It is important to note that Austin's use of the term *performance* is similar to that of later queer theorists, such as Judith Butler. These theorists use the term *performance* differently from the way it is used by Erving Goffman and scholars following his dramaturgical approach, in which performance means role-playing. In contrast to them, Austin is interested in the phenomenon in which saying words performs the action they describe. Austin's essay makes his own point that "utterances" (the words used to perform actions) are "successful" only within appropriate contexts: I could only perform his examples successfully if I were a mid-twentieth-century Englishman in the British civil service. (I was not.) For example, I could say "I name this ship the *Queen Elizabeth*," but the ship would not thereby be named the *Queen Elizabeth* because I, unfortunately, am not empowered to name British sailing vessels.

   I have found recent critiques and elaborations of Austin's theory of performance tremendously useful, particularly those dealing with medical anthropology (Martin, *Bipolar Expeditions*) and the study of economics (MacKenzie, Muniesa, and Siu, *Do Economists Make Markets?*). These scholars make the point that words accomplish tasks, and they develop the theory to show that successful performances depend on material artifacts, an argument that is implicit but underdeveloped in Austin's claim that the physical setting has to be right for utterances to be successful. MacKenzie argues this point particularly persuasively in chapter 3 of his coedited volume.

17. DiMaggio and Powell describe the phenomenon of "coercive isomorphism," in which organizations systematically adopt certain forms because of legal requirements. Powell and DiMaggio, introduction to *New Institutionalism*.

18. For important exceptions, see the following scholars, who have conducted ethnographies of IRBs and serve as inspiration for my work: Hedgecoe, "Research Ethics Review"; Jaeger, "Institutional Review Board Decision-Making"; Lederman, *Anthropology among the Disciplines*.

19. For critiques, see Bledsoe et al., "Regulating Creativity"; Dingwall, "Turn Off the Oxygen"; Feeley, "Legality, Social Research, and the Challenge of Institutional Review Boards"; Katz, "Toward a Natural History of Ethical Censorship"; Jacob and Riles, "New Bureaucracies of Virtue"; and Zachary M. Schrag, Institutional Review Blog, www.institutionalreviewblog.com. For a useful taxonomy of the IRB literature, see Heimer and Petty, "Bureaucratic Ethics," who suggest three categories of critique: law, regulation, and norms.

20. I occasionally accept invitations to sit in on meetings at other places for fun, I try to help researchers and board members recognize and manage the quirks of the review system, and I now volunteer on the IRB at a local community health clinic. I am fascinated by the claim that bureaucracies are tedious, in light of the fact that bureaucracies are made up of inherently interesting people.

21. *Final Report of the Advisory Committee*; Faden and Beauchamp, *History and Theory*; Frankel, "Human Experimentation in the United States"; Harkness, *Research behind Bars*; Kutcher, *Contested Medicine*, chap. 2; McCarthy, "Institutional Review Boards."

22. On the regional review system in the UK, see Hedgecoe, "Research Ethics Review." Some have proposed similar regional boards for the United States: e.g., Loh and Meyer, "Use of Central Institutional Review Boards"; Menikoff, "The Problem with Multiple-IRB Review"; Wagner et al., "Costs and Benefits"; Wood, Grady, and Emanuel, "Regional Ethics Organizations." Psychiatrist and ethicist Jay Katz was an early proponent of a nonlocal review system.

23. E.g., Annas and Grodin, *Nazi Doctors and the Nuremberg Code*; Brandt, "Racism and Research"; Goodman, McElligott, and Marks, *Useful Bodies*; Jones, *Bad Blood*; Reverby, *Examining Tuskegee*; Roelcke and Maio, *Twentieth Century Ethics of Human Subjects Research*.

24. Reverby, "'Normal Exposure' and Inoculation Syphilis."

25. Contra Rothman, *Strangers at the Bedside*. Both Cooter and Martensen develop this critique in persuasive essay reviews, which I follow here. Cooter, "Resistable Rise of Medical Ethics"; Martensen, "History of Bioethics."

PART ONE

1. Adams, Greenly, and Sander State are pseudonyms for my research sites.

2. For details on research methods, see the appendix. I must be spare in describing the board members and meeting locations to maintain anonymity. The regulations are available online through electronic versions of the Code of Federal Regulations and through the federal office that oversees human-subjects protections, the Office for Human Research Protections, www.hhs.gov/ohrp/humansubjects/guidance/45cfr46 .htm#46.109.

3. First, "exempt" studies are those that involve procedures, such as secondary data analysis and observation of public behavior, in which it would be impossible to identify the people involved or to "intervene" in their lives in any way. Second, "expedited" studies are those that IRB administrators think (usually based on the researchers' advice) present risks to participants that are no greater than what they would experience in their everyday lives, including risks to their privacy, psychological well-being, and physical health. Generally speaking, studies can be expedited if they involve certain types of research procedures, such as interviews and collections of small amounts of blood. However, the line between studies that can be expedited and those requiring full-board review hinges on distinctions regarding the nature of risk and vulnerability. IRBs do not consistently define risk either numerically (e.g.,

one in ten) or using probabilistic words (e.g., rarely), which people interpret quite differently, according psychological studies. For details on the complexity of operationalizing these terms, see Labott and Johnson, "Psychological and Social Risks"; Hamilton, "Some Precision Would Be Helpful"; Rector, "How Should We Communicate the Likelihood of Risks?"

4. Bosk, *What Would You Do?*

5. National Bioethics Advisory Commission, "Ethical and Policy Issues."

6. The stipulation that committees should include minorities was designed quite overtly to make local committees compliant with federal affirmative action requirements during the late 1960s and early 1970s. Generally speaking, advocates of affirmative action in that period challenged the idea that benefits accrued to investigators based on merit; those advocates argued instead that when an investigator's competence and integrity were taken into account, they were often unfairly intertwined with the person's ascribed traits. For the Department of Health, Education, and Welfare in particular in the early 1970s, it became an urgent priority to ensure equitable representation of race and gender in the membership of expert groups (IRBs and funding panels) operating under the department's aegis. The aim of the diversity clause introduced into IRB membership guidelines was as much to include members who could advocate for *investigators* belonging to a group that was traditionally discriminated against in science as it was to involve members that would advocate for human subjects who were minorities. In other words, the inclusion of women and minorities on review committees (on top of the existing categories of expert and layman) was intended in part to introduce an investigators' advocate. On this general point, which I am extending to IRBs, see Rossiter, *Women Scientists in America*.

7. These statistics are based on a study by De Vries and Forsberg. They took a novel and very useful approach in their survey by using "the IRB" as the unit of analysis rather than the IRB member. This allowed them to point out the homogeneity of many boards. Specifically, the authors found that of the 87 IRBs that responded to their survey, 28 percent had only white members and that 69 percent had a male majority. De Vries and Forsberg, "What Do IRBs Look Like?"

8. For most faculty members, serving on an IRB also filled a university service requirement, and depending on the institution and their role on the board, some members were compensated with stipends or with course release. At one university where faculty members' IRB stipends were calculated as a percentage of their base salaries, community members were given a flat-rate stipend; at another institution, the only members who received stipends were the board chair and one outside clinician. Those who had the smallest material incentive, but perhaps the greatest commitment, to serve on their IRB were the lay community members. They often cited as reasons for participating the personal reward of being able to discuss research with knowledgeable people and their personal commitment to serving (or fostering) "the community."

9. Brenneis, "Documenting Ethics." Lamont echoes this point in *How Professors Think*, 119–20.

10. The Belmont Report was the product of a commission mandated by the 1974 National Research Act, which also set human-subjects regulations in place. The Belmont principles are said to guide American research ethics and regulation. There are three principles: respect for persons, beneficence, and justice. In practice, these principles are brought to bear through IRB members' assessment of study risks, appropriateness of informed consent, and equity of subject selection. The Belmont Report is avail-

able online through the Office for Human Research Protections at http://ohsr.od.nih
.gov/guidelines/belmont.html.

11. Evans, "Growth of Principlism." The same year the Belmont Report was published, Beauchamp and Childress published the very influential *Principles of Biomedical Ethics*, in which they included their own set of principles, which are strikingly similar to the Belmont principles: autonomy, nonmaleficence, beneficence, and justice.

12. On balancing in the law, see Koch, *Administrative Law and Practice.*

13. Espeland and Vannebo, "Accountability, Quantification, and Law," 24. See also Centeno, "New Leviathan"; Stryker, "Rules, Resources, and Legitimacy Processes," 851.

14. Intramural Program, NIH, http://ohsr.od.nih.gov/guidelines/belmont.html; Amadae, *Rationalizing Capitalist Democracy*; Evans, *Playing God?*

15. SG, Aug.: 333, 362, 364.

16. SG, Aug.: 345. See the appendix for a list of transcription conventions.

17. Scott, *Seeing like a State.*

18. Jasanoff, "Science and the Statistical Victim."

19. SG, Oct.: 87. For an excellent analysis of how biological, legal, and social categories are mapped onto each other in research and its regulation, see Epstein, *Inclusion*. His study of clinical-trial recruitment requirements demonstrates how efforts to include categories of people in research in the name of equity—children as well as adults, women as well as men, and blacks as well as whites—have been regarded as positive moves toward pulling apart the generalizations on which social policy and medical therapies have been based. At the same time, the "inclusion" vigilance that the federal government requires of many IRBs also firms up such categories. Thus, IRBs are sites where it is possible to see how categories that are at the same time used as legal, social, and scientific groupings, such as race and gender, get locked together. The categorizations come together through small, nearly imperceptible choices, as in the case I described in which an IRB member requested a change to a study questionnaire that, in effect, would tell parents and children that reporting their race should make them feel uncomfortable.

20. SG, May: 501.

21. SG, Aug.: 255–61.

22. Ewick and Silbey, *Common Place of the Law.*

23. Boltanski and Thévenot have argued that readers of bureaucratic documents—in their case, surveys—unwittingly imagine the real people behind standard documents. This assessment of other people via documents is essential to the work of running a modern bureaucratic state; it is also how social biases are reproduced. See Boltanski and Thévenot, *On Justification.*

24. NG, July: 091, 399.

25. D2: 231.

26. D2: 271.

27. B7.

28. Med, July: 1 (paraphrased from field notes).

29. Guetzkow, Lamont, and Mallard, "What Is Originality?" The authors' analyses of funding-panel deliberations have shown that reviewers often infer an investigator's "scholastic virtues" from aspects of the proposal. In this way, reviewers inevitably make moral evaluations of investigators' character, which have been traditionally regarded as illegitimate biases in decision making, because indicators of investigators' character are inextricably linked with other criteria of evaluation. Typically, evaluations based on an investigator's nationality or native language, for example, are transgressions and cannot legitimately be used to assess investigators' scholastic

virtues, in the way that housekeeping work is used. On groups' speech norms, see Eliasoph and Lichterman, "Culture in Interaction"; Lamont, *How Professors Think*. The classic study of credibility production is Shapin and Schaffer, *Leviathan and the Air-Pump*. A large body of literature in science studies demonstrates the many ways in which trust and credibility have been generated and ritualized as a necessary part of the conduct of science.

30. Taylor and co-workers showed that when an IRB started requesting that researchers attend meetings, it took fewer meetings to approve studies and less correspondence between researchers and the IRB. While this piece of evidence based on a single board is by no means indisputable, the authors have solidly shown that investigators' presence at IRB meetings at least does not slow down approval: see Taylor, Currie, and Kass, "Effect of Investigator Attendance." See also Bell, Whiton, and Connelly, "Final Report," 37–38. The NIH commissioned the authors to conduct a survey of IRBs in which they compared low-volume and high-volume IRBs. They found that "42 percent of administrators from low-volume IRBs, compared to 17 percent from high-volume IRBs, noted that investigators were routinely encouraged to attend the meetings or to be reachable by telephone. . . . In contrast, 41 percent of administrators from high-volume IRBs, compared to 22 percent from low-volume IRBs, reported that investigators attended the meetings, or were on call, only when requested by the IRB."

31. Cerulo argues that Americans have better developed cognitive maps for projecting good scenarios for themselves than for projecting bad scenarios. She wrote this before the global financial crisis started in 2008, and since then she has reflected on the implications of this major historical unraveling for her theory of social cognition. Cerulo, *Never Saw It Coming*. By contrast, Sunstein argues that worst-case scenarios are more accessible to people when imagining the future. I do not take these arguments to be contradictory because they refer to different situations in which people are envisioning the future. Cerulo has in mind middle-class Americans thinking about their own lives. Sunstein, implicitly, is talking about government employees acting in their roles as agents of the state. See Sunstein, *Worst-Case Scenarios*.

CHAPTER ONE

1. SG, Oct.: 267.

2. See my "IRBs in Myth and Practice" and the other contributions to the December 2007 *Law and Society Review*. This issue is indicative of the fact that although many researchers say that IRBs do not have a legitimate claim to authority, researchers follow IRBs' requests anyway. It suggests that IRBs have power, even if it is not regarded as legitimate authority.

3. Guston, "On Consensus and Voting in Science"; Moreno, *Deciding Together*. IRB meetings are much like other government meetings in that people other than board members rarely attend. Irvin and Stansbury, "Citizen Participation in Decision Making."

4. Brenneis, "Documenting Ethics"; Reed, "Documents Unfolding"; Smith, "Incorporating Texts into Ethnographic Practice."

5. Gutmann, "Bureaucracy, Professionalism, and Participation," 209–11; Titunik, "Democracy, Domination, and Legitimacy."

6. Wuthnow, "Promoting Social Trust," 235; Wuthnow, "Trust as an Aspect of Social Structure"; Toulmin, "Layout of Arguments," 91–93.

7. Bernstein, *Class, Codes, and Control*, chap. 2, "A Public Language," 65–66.

8. Wuthnow, "Trust as an Aspect of Social Structure," 153–54, emphasis in original; see also Shapin, *Social History of Truth*; Eliasoph and Lichterman, "Culture in Interaction."
9. D5: 22–26.
10. B6: 32, 50.
11. Ibid.
12. For a history of the epistemic virtue of "objectivity," which has meant different things over the past four centuries, see Daston and Galison, *Objectivity*.
13. Collins and Evans, *Rethinking Expertise*, 22. See also Wynne, "May the Sheep Safely Graze?"; Epstein, *Impure Science*; Rabeharisoa and Callon, "Patients and Scientists"; Shapin, "Trusting George Cheyne"; Williams and Popay, "Lay Knowledge."
14. NG, June: 144.
15. C6: 331.
16. C6: 331.
17. Polletta, *It Was like a Fever*; Polletta and Lee, "Telling Stories."
18. For update information on child-abuse reporting laws, see the U.S. Administration for Children and Families' online Child Welfare Information Gateway.
19. SG, June: 324–25.
20. NG, July: 350.
21. NG, July: 350.
22. NG, July: 373.
23. NG, July: 383.
24. Guetzkow, Lamont, and Mallard, "What Is Originality?"
25. An excellent overview of the literature on tacit knowledge and embodied skill is Shapin and Lawrence, "Body of Knowledge."
26. SG, Nov.: 864.
27. SG, Nov.: 970.
28. SG, Nov.: 896.
29. Shapin, "Trusting George Cheyne." Likewise, Polletta has shown that among members of civic groups, personal stories can move groups toward consensus. *Freedom Is an Endless Meeting*, chap. 6; Polletta, *It Was like a Fever*; Polletta and Lee, "Telling Stories."
30. Brown, "Fairly Balanced," 549.
31. See, e.g., Williams and Popay, "Lay Knowledge"; Durant, "Accounting for Expertise," 5.
32. On the general problem of access for empirical research on regulation, see Espeland and Vannebo, "Accountability, Quantification, and Law." For examples, see Jasanoff, *Designs on Nature*; Kevles, *Baltimore Case*; Carpenter, *Reputation and Power*.
33. Thorpe and Shapin, "Who Was Oppenheimer?"; Porter, *Trust in Numbers*; Timmermans, *Postmortem*.
34. Bernstein, *Class, Codes, and Control*, 63.
35. Attention to warrants is a particularly useful way to explain decisions among peer groups. Organizational sociologists have fruitfully studied groups that have a vertical structure—that have, in other words, a formal hierarchy among members, such as bosses and subordinates: e.g., Stevens, *Creating a Class*; Vaughn, *Challenger Launch Decision*, chap. 8. In these cases, decisions are generally attributed to the power structure of the group. Based on this empirical literature, it is difficult to explain how decisions are made in groups without an obvious vertical structure, particularly in groups characterized by what Polletta calls "complex equality," in which all participants are considered equally valuable but valuable for very different reasons. *Freedom Is an*

Endless Meeting, chap. 6. (Here Polletta fruitfully appropriates Michael Walzer's term, which he originally used to theorize resource allocation.) Thus, the study of warrants is a way to analyze decision making in groups like IRBs that have a more horizontal structure, often by design.

36. Lee, "Private Conversation in Public Dialogue"; Polletta, *Freedom Is an Endless Meeting,* chap. 6; Wilde, *Vatican II,* chap. 3.

CHAPTER TWO

1. "These results suggest a 'two strikes and you're out' mentality among employers who appear to view the combination of blackness and criminal record as an indicator of serious trouble," writes Devah Pager, a researcher exploring how racism magnifies the negative effects of crime in the United States. "Where for whites, a criminal background represents one serious strike against them, for blacks it appears to represent almost total disqualification." Pager, *Marked,* 146–47.

2. Fisher, *Medical Research for Hire*; Loh and Meyer, "Use of Central Institutional Review Boards"; Menikoff, "The Problem with Multiple-IRB Review"; Petryna, *When Experiments Travel.*

3. For details on the methodology, see the appendix. Two of my twenty interviews ran long, so I had to cut the question about the standard protocol. I am reporting here the responses of eighteen IRB chairs. One shortcoming of studies of IRBs using standard protocols, including the audit studies I reviewed, as well as my own interview questions, is that these studies often erase the markers (e.g., a researcher's identity) that are instrumental in helping IRBs judge protocols. That is to say, standard-protocol studies are somewhat contrived and do not conform to the way boards usually encounter protocols.

4. N18: 66.

5. N8: 134.

6. I told the board chairs I interviewed that this hypothetical protocol was based on a real study that had been published recently in the *American Journal of Sociology.* To minimize confusion, I left out the additional independent variable of incarceration, which accentuates but does not change the finding of racial discrimination. The researcher has since expanded that study into a book, cited in note 1. During the interviews, I asked the chairs to read the protocol; in phone interviews, I read it to them.

7. Code of Federal Regulation, 45 CFR 46.116, general requirements for informed consent, section d: "An IRB may approve a consent procedure which does not include, or which alters, some or all of the elements of informed consent set forth in this section, or waive the requirements to obtain informed consent provided the IRB finds and documents that: (1) The research involves no more than minimal risk to the subjects; (2) The waiver or alteration will not adversely affect the rights and welfare of the subjects; (3) The research could not practicably be carried out without the waiver or alteration; and (4) Whenever appropriate, the subjects will be provided with additional pertinent information after participation." There are other rules that pertain to research on medical interventions. For a history of the role of psychology in inserting this caveat during the 1970s, see Stark, "The Science of Ethics."

8. N2: 338.

9. B4: 56.

10. N1: 643–51.

11. B4: 56.

12. N6: 180.
13. N11: 111.
14. N16: 158.
15. N14: 244.
16. N15: 250.
17. N16: 166.
18. One of the earliest IRB audit studies looked at thirty-two boards and concluded that many of the disparate changes that IRBs requested compromised the scientific integrity of the research design. Goldman and Katz, "Inconsistency and Institutional Review Boards." For evidence of differences in IRB decisions and a discussion of the implications for multisite studies, see Burman et al., "Effects of Local Review"; Silverman, Hull, and Sugarman, "Variability among Decisions"; McWilliams et al., "Problematic Variation"; Green et al., "Impact of Variation"; Hirshon et al., "Variability in Assessment"; Stair et al., "Variation in Responses." For an overview of the special frustrations with IRB variation expressed by investigators conducting minimal-risk research, see Ernst et al., "Minimal-Risk Waiver"; Green et al., "Impact of Variation."
19. Each of these threads has a vast literature. Broadly speaking, on the issue of local cultures and epistemologies, I have in mind small-group studies among cultural sociologists, such as Gary Alan Fine's work on idioculture (e.g., "Sociology of the Local") and lab studies in the field of science and technology. Debates around path dependency have been most fruitfully set loosely in historical-comparative studies in political sociology.
20. NG, Feb.: 553.
21. NG, Dec.: 136.
22. NG, Feb.: 433.
23. SG, Apr.: 154.
24. SG, May: 255.
25. SG, May: 303–23. Words in parentheses were inaudible on the audio recording and are taken from field notes of the meeting.
26. SG, May.
27. SG, May: 361–63.
28. SG, June: 86–92.
29. Hacking, *Historical Ontology*. Though for a critique of Hacking's "styles of scientific reasoning," see Kusch, "Hacking's Historical Epistemology."
30. Forrester, "If p, Then What?" 21. See also Forrester, "Psychoanalytic Case."
31. Kuhn, *Structure of Scientific Revolutions*. Forrester likewise describes reasoning in cases as central to the philosophy of science of his mentor, T. S. Kuhn, for whom "one learns to do science not by learning the rules or principles or concepts and then applying them to concrete situations; rather, one learns how to do science by learning how to work the exemplars: extending them, reproducing them, turning a novel situation into a version of a well-understood exemplar." Forrester, "If p, Then What?" 7.
32. Eliasoph and Lichterman, "Culture in Interaction."
33. Heimer, "Cases and Biographies," 56. Heimer understands cases in law and medicine somewhat differently from how they are understood by Kuhn and Forrester, who are interested in how new instances are compared back to a particularly important case that has been given a higher status than all others. Heimer, by contrast, thinks of cases as being more like links in a chain, where people move from one to the next, nonetheless dealing with each link in a very similar way. On the particular question

of qualitative review, I agree with the view presented in Hedgecoe, "Research Ethics Review."

34. Personal communication, March 19, 2010.

CHAPTER THREE

1. SG, Nov.: 987–92.
2. Waddell, "Reasonableness versus Rationality"; Brenneis, "Discourse and Discipline"; Tsay et al., "From Character to Intellect"; Guetzkow, Lamont, and Mallard, "What Is Originality?"; Lamont, *How Professors Think*; Lamont and Huutoniemi, "Customary Rules of Fairness"; Lederman, *Anthropology among the Disciplines*; Wood, "Sociologies of Knowledge"; Stevens, *Creating a Class*, chap. 6.
3. Law, "On STS and Sociology," see esp. 635; McKenzie, Muniesa, and Siu, *Do Economists Make Markets?*
4. Weber, *Economy and Society*, 219.
5. Code of Federal Regulation, 45 CFR 46.115.
6. Suchman, "Contract as Social Artifact."
7. For examples, see Foucault, *Discipline and Punish*; Hacking, "Making Up People"; Heimer, "Cases and Biographies"; Igo, *Averaged American*; Rose, *Inventing Ourselves*; Shore and Wright, "Coercive Accountability"; Timmermans and Berg, *Gold Standard*.
8. Garfinkel, *Studies in Ethnomethodology*, 200.
9. Ibid., 197.
10. Reed, "Documents Unfolding"; Smith, "Incorporating Texts into Ethnographic Practice."
11. Taylor, Currie, and Kass, "Effect of Investigator Attendance."
12. SG, Nov.: 631.
13. SG, Nov.: 857.
14. SG, Nov.: 865–66.
15. For more on what I call the warranting process in IRB meetings, see chapter 1. In short, IRB members tended to justify their views in three main ways: by invoking their professional experience (such as having researched a similar group of people), their private experience (such as having cared for their own sick child), and publicly available matters of fact (such as knowing the most recent demographics of a neighborhood). Board members tended to find a justification based on professional experience most persuasive because it represented, by definition, both uncommon and expert knowledge and thus was difficult to contest.
16. SG, Nov.: 906.
17. SG, Nov.: 953.
18. SG, Nov.: 872.
19. SG, Nov.: 878.
20. SG, Nov.: 970.
21. SG, Nov.: 906–13.
22. SG, Nov.: 879–913.
23. SG, Nov.: 895–902.
24. SG, Nov.: 951.
25. SG, Nov.: 987–92.
26. NG, April: 241.
27. NG, April: 245.
28. NG, April: 246.
29. Researchers must also follow the Health Insurance Portability and Accountability

Act's Privacy and Security Rules, through the Department of Health and Human Services' Office of Civil Rights.

30. NG, April: 606–15.

31. NG, April: 620.

32. Brenneis, "Discourse and Discipline."

33. NG, April: 630.

34. NG, April: 71, 342–43.

35. Austin, *How to Do Things with Words*; Latour, *Science in Action*; Shapin, *Social History of Truth*.

36. Smith, "Incorporating Texts into Ethnographic Practice."

PART TWO

1. There have been a few exceptions: NIH was given regulatory responsibility for stem cell research in 2009. In addition, the predecessor to the Office for Human Research Protections (OHRP), which regulates IRBs today, was originally located within NIH and on the Bethesda campus. Part of the justification for moving the OHRP out of NIH physically and organizationally was that NIH should not be responsible for research regulation because the agency sponsored research. Today, NIH itself is regulated by OHRP and other regulatory agencies, such as the Food and Drug Administration, which regulates drugs and devices. For an excellent political history of the FDA, see Carpenter, *Reputation and Power*. NIH has its own intramural IRB. See Fletcher, "Location of the Office."

2. There are ancillary locations for the Intramural Program, including the offices just north of the main campus in Rockville, and some institutes have facilities in other states.

3. Stark and Theodorou, "Hospital Architecture."

4. Topping, "Clinical Center for Medical Research." For an example of growing dissatisfaction with the intellectual division between clinical and laboratory medicine two decades earlier, see Luckhardt's 1923 article "The Progress of Medicine," which is cited in Geison, "Divided We Stand." Despite the unification of clinical and laboratory research, at an administrative level the categorical institutes were still separate, so there were continual problems in coordinating shared resources, such as nursing staff, and the problems were compounded by the organization of the institutes around disease categories (the style of organization Congress insisted upon) rather than around research areas. Mandel, "Beacon of Hope."

5. Nathan, "Careers in Translational Clinical Research"; Schechter, "Crisis in Clinical Research." The early leaders of the Clinical Center disagreed about whether the facility should be called a hospital, given the research orientation. The organization and by-laws committee appeared to have "made certain assumptions as to the similarity in the administrative structure of NIH to the administrative organization of a hypothetical hospital. The purpose of this was to set forth the administrative organization in such a way that it would be understood by accrediting bodies as well as the staff. . . . In addition, there was objection voiced to referring to the Clinical Center as a hospital." They did finally decide it was a hospital, but this dispute reveals the unsettled status of studying people in a clinical settings. Medical Board meeting minutes, November 23, 1953, minutes, box 1, folder "Minutes of the Medical Board Jan 6 1953–May 1954," Med Board, NIH.

6. Strickland, *Politics, Science, and Dread Disease*, 174; Kanigel, *Apprentice to Genius*, 24.

7. For "golden age" reminiscences, see Park, "Intramural Research Program."

8. Memo to the heads of institutions conducting research with Public Health Service Grants from the Surgeon General, February 8, 1966, folder 2, Ethical, Moral, and Legal Aspects, CC, ONIHH, NIH.
9. See my "IRBs in Myth and Practice." Schrag, in *Ethical Imperialism* and in "Talking Became Human Subjects Research," also explains how the regulations developed in terms of the social sciences.
10. McCarthy explains that James Shannon's September 28, 1965, statement to the National Advisory Health Council that introduced the policy the surgeon general announced five months later was, in the history of ethics, "a significant historical change that went almost unnoticed at the time. . . . The policy that Shannon recommended to the NAHC in 1965 borrowed and expanded the Clinical Center policy to all research subjects involved in both intramural and extramural research." McCarthy, "Institutional Review Boards."

CHAPTER FOUR

1. The names of all of the healthy patients in this book are pseudonyms. Quotations and details on individual Normal patients come from their patient records, housed in MRD, NIH. The NIH Office of Human Subjects Research granted me permission to see the records of selected patients and to cite the records, so long as I did not include personal identifiable information (such as social security numbers and birthdays) or private health information. It is worth noting that "cooperation" was the trait that researchers most coveted in patients, perhaps more than perfect physical health. NIH medical charts suggest this, especially when read along with other histories of research subjects; see, e.g., Prescott, "Using the Student Body," 9. The Normal Volunteer Patient Program in 1960 specifically "appraised" Normal volunteers based on their "cooperation, interest, and attitude." Memo, May 25, 1960, requested by Maginnis per Himmelsbach, PRPL. For thoughtful reflections on the ethical and scholarly possibilities of using patient records in historical research, see Risse and Warner, "Reconstructing Clinical Activities." As these authors anticipated, privacy laws and popular sensibilities have changed in the past two decades, and it will continue to be difficult to predict how readers, publishers, and lawmakers will view the use of patient charts as historical sources.
2. Zimmerman record, MRD, NIH.
3. Abadie, *Professional Guinea Pig*; Elliott, "Guinea-Pigging"; Elliott and Abadie, "Exploiting a Research Underclass"; Dresser, "First-in-Human Trial Participants." See Stark and Kelly, Review of *Professional Guinea Pig*. It is revealing of the size and sustained engagement of research volunteers that there is a magazine, *Guinea Pig Zero*, whose target audience is human subjects. There is also a large body of literature that critiques and analyzes the moral and financial market for human subjects. Standouts include Fisher, *Medical Research for Hire*; Petryna, *When Experiments Travel*. These books impressively document how research on new medical therapies often reproduces the social inequalities that health research would ideally alleviate. Current research regulations allow for-profit companies to create a market for new drugs while enrolling as subjects people whose health care tends to be the worst and their need for compensation the greatest. For-profit drug development does not fix, and may in fact exploit, gaps in medical infrastructures.

NIH leaders have long recognized the importance of word choice, and some started to press clinicians to use the term *volunteer* to refer to Normals starting around

1958. In one clinical staff meeting, for example, Dr. Joseph Smadel, the associate director for intramural research, tried to lead by example: "All through the discussion this afternoon I shall probably use the word 'volunteer' and except to identify these with the term that is frequently used here of 'normal control' or 'subject' I shall never use those words again. I feel very strongly about this, and I think perhaps if you used the word 'volunteer' a little more often, and less often talked about 'normal controls' and 'subjects' that you might approach this matter with a little more sensitivity than is derived from the word 'subject.'" Transcript of quarterly clinical staff meeting, January 9, 1958, LOC INTRA 2-1-A, ODEF, NIH. At the Clinical Center today, the metric used to determine payment is the "inconvenience unit." Scores of healthy volunteers are admitted to the Clinical Center each year. The following data on health volunteers at the NIH Clinical Center, giving number of visits by year of discharge, are from a personal e-mail communication, February 9, 2010, MRD, NIH. I thank Lauren Feld for organizing the data in this form. Note that one volunteer can have multiple visits; each readmission is counted as a new visit.

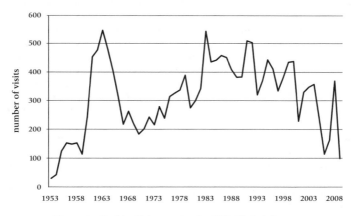

Figure 6a. Healthy Volunteers at the NIH Clinical Center.

4.   Outside of hospital walls, citizens including students, family members, and friends were used in laboratory research in medicine and social sciences. Lederer, *Subjected to Science*; Prescott, "Using the Student Body." These citizens were often subservient and open to coercion but were not members of what we would today call captive or institutionalized populations, such as prisoners, soldiers, and orphans. See Goodman et al., *Useful Bodies*; Washington, *Medical Apartheid* (for a more rounded, if limited, view on the use of slaves, see Emanuel, "Unequal Treatment," a review of *Medical Apartheid*; and Schiebinger, "Human Experimentation"). Historians argue that friends, family members, and students were used not only because they were convenient (which of course also factored, though documenting exploitation tends to muscle out other worthwhile questions in the historical literature). Historians have shown that scientists used these additional groups because they felt their closest companions gave more useful accounts of how they felt—precisely because these people tended to be better educated and part of the scientists' social milieu and local culture. Thus, choice of human subjects reflected scientists' concerns about good

communication as well as the practical matter of their convenience. This also suggests the paradox inherent in researchers' goal of creating objective medical knowledge that is itself dependent on subjective accounts of how people feel.

5. On the negative moral valences of intervening in the lives of healthy people before World War II, see DeHue, "History of the Control Group." On the changing function of American hospitals over the nineteenth and twentieth centuries, see Rosenberg, *Care of Strangers*; Starr, *Social Transformation of American Medicine*, book 1, chap. 4; Stevens, *In Sickness and in Wealth*. On how normal control patients strained doctors' rhetoric of safeguarding people through the doctor-patient relationship, see McCarthy, "Institutional Review Boards," 543. Charles McCarthy was the first director of the Office for Protection from Research Risks, the forerunner to the current federal Office for Human Research Protections, which oversees the Code of Federal Regulation, 45 CFR 46. Culling through his personal notes from the period, McCarthy wrote that in the early 1950s, "most NIH investigators conducting research involving humans still thought of themselves as medical practitioners. Clinical Center officials argued that it would be an unjustified intrusion into the doctor-patient relationship to allow any administrative body to interfere with the relationship between physician/investigator and their research subjects/patients. Nevertheless, even those who held this view recognized that this argument could not be made with respect to normal volunteers—that is, healthy people who volunteered to serve as research subjects." See also Frankel, "Human Experimentation in the United States."

6. On debate about moving a patient, see Medical Board meeting minutes, March 10, 1964; and on discussion of the "threshold" of the Clinical Center, see Medical Board meeting minutes, November 12, 1964, both in box 1, folder Medical Board meeting minutes, February 12, 1963–September 22, 1964, Med Board, NIH.

7. Medical Board meeting minutes, June 9, 1953, box 1, folder "Minutes Jan 6 1953–May 1954," Med Board, NIH.

8. Harkness, *Research behind Bars*, 152; Lederer, "Research without Borders." In 2007 the Institute of Medicine recommended that lawmakers ease the regulations binding research in prisons, a position that drew heavy criticism. Gostin et al., *Ethical Considerations*.

9. Wyatt, "Commentary." NIH was not a defendant in the relevant lawsuit, but the intramural researchers were doing virus studies at the same site and collaborating with extramural researchers at the University of Maryland who were defendants. Documents from the lawsuit are published in Gilchrist and Urban Information Interpreters, *Medical Experimentation on Prisoners*.

10. For a masterful history of the FDA and its weaknesses as a regulatory agency, see Carpenter, *Reputation and Power*. Other historians document how the regulations were weakened by lack of funding for enforcement and by the influence of industry figures who were paraded as outside experts. See, e.g., Tobbell, "Allied against Reform." For an excellent internal account, see Junod, "History of Informed Patient Consent." On the mixed results of polio vaccine testing and manufacture, see Marks, "Salk Poliomyelitis Vaccine Field Trial"; Offit, *Cutter Incident*. Stevens has argued that the well-known success of pharmaceuticals during World War II, which happened quickly and with government coordination of clinical trials, affirmed the importance of science for healing patients and, in turn, the importance of hospital-based laboratories for clinical science. Stevens, *In Sickness and in Wealth*, chap. 8.

11. Creager, "Molecular Surveillance"; Creager, "Nuclear Energy." See the companion articles included in the special issue "Radiobiology in the Atomic Age" of the *Journal of the History of Biology* in 2006. See also Jones and Martensen, "Human Radiation

Experiments." The authors show that radiation research was a national priority in the 1940s and 1950s, using the case of San Francisco research institutions. Their main aim is to argue that a good deal of research on sick patients was "transgressive" even by the standards of the medical profession at the time but that actors had interests in creating a new field of medical physics and advancing their own careers. The authors reemphasize interest-driven history and argue that histories that hedge over wrongdoing or fall back on historical relativism are too forgiving. Those authors would share this view with like-minded historians Jay Katz and Paul Weindling. On nuclear medicine at NIH, see "Studies on Radiation Biology." A radiation lab occupied three floors below ground and five floors above ground at the Clinical Center. According to that article in the *NIH Record*, the aim was to "provide facilities for the application of discoveries in the new field of nuclear energy, including the radioactive isotopes." The article continued, "This wing will contain 20 beds for patients needing short-term radiation treatment. The center will be exceptionally well equipped to conduct nuclear energy research." The equipment included a 12-million-volt electrostatic generator, a synchrotron, and a 2-million-volt radiotherapy machine. "A staff thoroughly trained in the use of radiation under strictly controlled conditions will use this and other equipment for laboratory research, treatment of patients, and preparation of radioactive substances to be used for both treatment and research." Already in 1953, radiation measurement was a strong suit at NIH. A radioactive switchboard from another clinic was transported to NIH for testing at the Isotope Lab. Afterward, the switchboard was encased in concrete, handed off to the Coast Guard, and thrown overboard into the Atlantic Ocean somewhere off the coast of Norfolk, Virginia. "NIH Experts Test Switchboard."

12. Terrill to Kidd, NIH chief of research planning, September 25, 1950, box S09F01B0087, folder 18, Series: Research Collections, Advisory Committee on Human Radiation Experiments, RG 220, NARAII. See the contents of this box for interactions between NIH and other members of the Department of Defense circa 1950.

13. "Practice Runs Show Progress," in the 1952 "Civil Defense" issue of the *NIH Record* recounts and offers points after the second dry run. It states, "To make our tactical problem as simple as possible we are assuming an atomic explosion in downtown Washington during work hours" (1).

14. Drug research and nuclear medicine were related because scientists were able to see the effects of chemical molecules when they were tagged with radioisotopes. For an excellent primer on radiation research, see "The Basics of Radiation Research," in *The Final Report of the Advisory Committee on Human Radiation Experiments*, 43–68. On the history of research methods in drug research, see Marks, "Trust and Mistrust." The foundational text is Marks, *The Progress of Experiment*. Marks argued that the adoption of randomized controlled trials as the gold standard in medical evidence was fueled in the 1930s by activists, who were alarmed by the doctors' exuberant and untracked use of the many new drugs on the market. Our adoption of randomized controlled trials in the present day was not driven, he argues, by doctors' slowly realizing that randomized controlled trials were a superior method for establishing safety and efficacy, but rather by doctors' bending to reformers' demands and overcoming problems of coordination between disparate locations.

15. Goodman, McElligott, and Marks, *Useful Bodies*; Guerrini, "Human Rights, Animal Rights"; Harkness, *Research behind Bars*; Moreno, *Undue Risk*.

16. The Atomic Energy Commission regulated the shipping of radioisotopes and granted authorization to researchers in particular places. Creager, "Nuclear Energy"; Richard Riseberg, legal adviser, NIH, to Sidney Edelman, assistant general counsel for PHS,

Subject: LSD Research, April 7, 1976, box 26, folder "Gov Rel 2–10 NIH-CIA MK-ULTRA project, 1976–79," NIH Central Files, Office of Director, RG 443, NARAII (finding aid: UD-06D, RG 443: 130: 53: 11: 4–6).

17. For every patient bed in the Clinical Center, there were two laboratory modules to go with it. Transcript of quarterly clinical staff meeting, January 9, 1958, LOC INTRA 2-1-A, ODEF, NIH.

18. Zimmerman record, MRD, NIH.

19. Fahrenthold, "It's a Model Hospital."

20. Haseltine, "Hospital Primarily for Research"; transcript of quarterly clinical staff meeting, January 9, 1958, LOC INTRA 2-1-A, ODEF, NIH.

21. "Patient Reaction to CC Is Reported in Survey," *NIH Record* 6, no. 21 (November 29, 1954).

22. Scientists' Committee on Loyalty and Security, "Loyalty and Service Grants." For secondary accounts, see Wang, *American Science*, 280; Caute, *Great Fear*, 472. Pauling had been working on developing artificial blood, a project that previously had been funded by HEW. In 1956 HEW announced that it had changed its policy of loyalty criteria for awarding funds. Nonetheless, in 1969 it was discovered that HEW had continued to blacklist researchers who seemed to be politically subversive, and in response there was general uproar among American researchers. See, for example, the contents of s17, box 88, folder "1970 Federal Funding," AAA.

23. Transcript of quarterly clinical staff meeting, January 9, 1958, LOC INTRA 2-1-A, p. 9, ODEF, NIH.

24. Jack Masur was the first and also the third director of the Clinical Center. During a brief interlude, Patrick Trautman was the director. Masur had been assigned a different position in the PHS, but owing to his unhappiness with the office job and his skill directing the hospital, he was allowed to resume directorship of the Clinical Center. Henry Masur, personal communication, 2009.

25. Hillyer to Siepert (through Masur, copies to Ladimer and Rourke), April 6, 1951, LOC INTRA 2-1-A, ODEF, NIH. Hillyer and Ladimer had previously spoken about NIH legislation "needs." Rourke to Masur, May 24, 1951, LOC INTRA 2-1-A, ODEF, NIH.

26. For an overall sense of the total work of the Office of General Counsel for NIH, including Rourke's tasks, see the contents of box 1, folder 14, 1952 (DHEW), Office of General Counsel, Public Health Division, Records Relating to Actions and Advice of the General Counsel, 1951–69, RG 235, NARAII (finding aid: A1, entry 33-C: 130: 66: 42).

27. Masur to Rourke, January 8, 1951; Rourke to Masur, May 24, 1951, LOC INTRA 2-1-A, ODEF, NIH. In his reply to Masur's questions, Rourke wrote, "As to care during the period of study, we believe in general that you would be authorized to maintain the health of the patient to the degree enjoyed by him upon his admission in order to assure his continued usefulness to, or his cooperation in, the study. For example, disease contracted after admission even though nonemergency and not of direct significance to the study, could be treated if such treatment contributed either maintain the patients' usefulness to, or qualification for, the study, or he being in any event so useful or qualified, such treatment reasonably contributed to his continued participation. As to the latter, we gather that the loss to the study of a single case reduces the efficiency and perhaps the effectiveness of the project so that treatment for assuring continued participation may be on this basis alone important to the study function. The point at which it would be preferable to discharge the patient as one no longer appropriate for study, or to supply him care to assure his continued participation would be a matter for medical judgment."

28. Halisky, "Church Volunteers"; Haseltine, "Objectors Aid Health Tests."

29. Bert C record, MRD, NIH. All quotes from Social Services are from volunteers' records.

30. I. Ladimer, "Normal Volunteer Participation in Clinical Research," April 12, 1954, PRPL, NIH.

31. Zimmerman record, MRD, NIH. NIH expected the biggest problem for Normals would be "boredom." See "Normal Volunteers."

32. Transcript of quarterly clinical staff meeting, January 9, 1958, LOC INTRA 2-1-A, p. 24, ODEF, NIH.

33. Medical Board meeting minutes, May 11, 1954, box 1, folder 3, RG 443/CC, NARAII.

34. For a detailed contemporary record of World War II alternative service programs, including locations for Program Guinea Pig, see Gingerich, *Service for Peace*. For accounts of Ancel Keyes's research on conscientious objectors at the University of Minnesota, which give careful consideration to how religious understanding of service and sacrifice intersect with scientists' demands, see Tucker, *Great Starvation Experiment*; Tracy, "Fasting for Research and Relief." For oral histories from religious objectors on various assignments during World War II, see Frazer and O'Sullivan, *Just Begun to Not Fight*.

35. Visscher, University of Minnesota, to Lewis Weed, October 12, 1940, Military Medicine File, folder: Committee on Medicine: Subcom: Clinical Investigation, 1940–42, NAS.

36. Mandel, "Beacon of Hope."

37. It is worth noting that Terry, a native of Alabama, was named after a family friend and local surgeon who was the father of the U.S. senator Lister Hill, himself credited (or blamed) for exorbitant federal funding provided to NIH during the 1950s and 1960s. This plausible justification for deciding to name a child Luther Leonidas is explained in Mullan, *Plagues and Politics*, 146.

38. Brandt, *Cigarette Century*.

39. Frazer and O'Sullivan, *Just Begun to Not Fight*; Gingerich, *Service for Peace*. Guinea Pig Projects were relatively small units (only 116 objectors were placed), and they started in the fourth year of American involvement in the war. The men considered the units to be tough assignments—and thus authentic service to the nation worth respecting and feeling proud of—on par with the "fire jumpers." In 1953, when NIH was negotiating to get religious objectors, the Mennonite Central Committee's Daniel Graber sent Ladimer a copy of Gingerich's *Service for Peace*, telling him, "A brief description of the guinea pig project appears on page 270. I am sure that will be of particular interest to you." Two weeks later, Ladimer thanked Graber for Gingerich's book. Graber to Ladimer, September 29, 1953; Ladimer to Graber, October 12, 1953, folder National Institutes of Health, 1954, MCA correspondence, IX-6-3, MCA.

40. Shannon to Loeb, November 10, 1944, NAS-DMS folder: Board for Coordination of Malarial Studies: Panels: Clinical Testing: Testing Centers: NYU: Goldwater Memorial Hospital, General, NAS. An attachment explains procedures for research and describes Goldwater's triumph of "selling" the malaria studies to subjects before "giving fever." The attachment was written by C. Gordon Zubrod, who had previously trained at Berkeley (see Heilbron and Seidel, *Lawrence and His Laboratory*) and later followed Shannon to NIH. This folder contains extensive lab notes, including lists of patients, drugs, and dosages used in trials (especially by Shannon acolyte and future NIH clinician Robert Berliner).

41. Shannon to R. Loeb, November 10, 1944. On esteem for Shannon among his contemporaries, see Loeb to Sheehan, June 16, 1944; Carden to Keefer, October 4, 1944, all three in NAS-MED folder: MED: Board for Coordination of Malarial Studies: Panels:

Clinical Testing: Testing Centers: NYU: Goldwater Memorial Hospital, General, NAS. See also Kennedy, "James Augustine Shannon," 9–10.

42. Kennedy, "James Augustine Shannon."

43. For Shannon's budgets, see "Goldwater Memorial Hospital 1945 Personnel Budget," NAS-MDS Board for Coordination of Malarial Studies: Panels: Clinical Testing: Folder: Reports to Board 1945, NAS. In addition, pay for conscientious objectors in malaria research was funded through the budgets of Massachusetts General Hospital and the University of Chicago. In addition to receiving U.S. Office of Scientific Research and Development funding for Goldwater research, Shannon was funded as director of the Central Unit for the Rockefeller Institute under Cassius Van Slyke (who was the first director of NIH's National Heart Institute). See the contents of the folder "Reports to Board 1945," Rockefeller Institute, Proposal for extension of contract, February 8, 1945. For general information on Shannon's research and oversight of malaria vaccine trials, see Shannon, "Clinical Testing of Antimalarial Drugs"; Kennedy, "James Augustine Shannon," 7–8. It is worth noting that Shannon had his conscientious objectors sign consent forms, which was customary when researchers studied soldiers.

44. For Shannon's desk copies of malaria trials and detailed patient results, see contents of box 19, folder 3: "Therapeutic Trials of Antimalarial Agents, Summary of charts, Research service, Third New York University Medical Division, Goldwater Memorial Hospital, Welfare Island, New York," MS C 363, James A. Shannon Papers, NLM, NIH. In his hagiographic account of postwar NIH researchers, Kanigel reflects on his work that Shannon oversaw at Green Haven. It was "an army prison whose inmates had volunteered to be injected with malarial blood. ('We asked them to volunteer, but I guess there was some implied reward, [Thomas] Kennedy admits')." Kanigel, *Apprentice to Genius*, 26. Waxing nostalgic at the end of the book, Kanigel observes: "Today, the conscientious objectors and prison inmates of the war years have given way to army volunteers and civilians, in some cases paid fifteen hundred dollars to suffer the chills and fever dealt out by the *Plasmodium* parasite" (244).

45. It is not clear who invited whom. The NIH account is that by coincidence Curry contacted NIH the same week that clinicians decided they should contact him.

46. Whedon is credited for the idea of the Normal Volunteers Patient Program, although it seems more likely that he was part of the New York set of drug researchers under Shannon's purview during World War II. Although Whedon's protocol served as the test case, Shannon's former home institute, National Heart Institute, actually got the first Normals.

47. Zimmerman record, MRD, NIH.

48. Transcript of quarterly clinical staff meeting, January 9, 1958, LOC INTRA 2-1-A, p. 23, ODEF, NIH.

49. "'Guinea Pig' Society." The article explains that the new "honor society" was open "only to scientists and laymen who have contributed to medical science as volunteer experimental subjects. Purpose of the new society is to provide recognition for contributions to medical progress." See also Harkness, *Research behind Bars*, 159. Harkness observes that prisoners were not allowed to join the club.

50. Patient record, MRD, NIH.

51. Folder: National Institutes of Health, 1954, MCA correspondence, IX-6-3, MCA. See also Haseltine, "Objectors Aid Health Tests." Ladimer wrote that he would "arrange procurement of volunteers" for NIH. Ladimer to Shannon, May 13, 1953, ODEF, NIH. Ladimer also discussed with Shannon the purchasing arrangement after

Ladimer and Dr. Whedon met with representatives of the National Board for Religious Objectors, including Curry, in mid-September 1953. Ladimer told Shannon, "[I] proposed arrangements under which I felt we could 'purchase' service from the organization on a man-month basis." Ladimer reported that the representatives "received the proposal very well and agreed to cooperate." Ladimer to Shannon, September 21, 1953, file LOC INTRA 2-1-A, ODEF, NIH. I would encourage researchers to seek out the rich contents of the Office of Director Electronic Files (ODEF, NIH). A similar-sounding physical holding is at the National Library of Medicine, but it appears to have been heavily processed: NIH Directors' Files, 1937–1983 (MS C 536), NLM, NIH.

52. In one meeting a church representative asked "what responsibility NIH [had] in the event of illness or death developing from research." Ladimer said, "Although this matter was not actually spelled out in the contracts, it is understood that we will take care of anything that developed directly from research here. With respect to what happens off duty, there is some question. If we release them [patients] inappropriately, as when under the influence of a drug, we would probably be responsible; otherwise not." The church then "agreed that they might take out insurance against this latter contingency." April 12, 1954, PRPL, NIH.

53. "Normal Volunteers." For Medical Board discussions of the Normals program, see Medical Board meeting minutes, October 13, 1953, box 1, folder 3, "Meeting minutes, 1952–4," RG 443/CC, NARAII. These minutes are duplicated in Medical Board meeting minutes at NLM, NIH.

54. Ladimer to Shannon, January 21, 1954. Ladimer encouraged Shannon to check up on the approval status of the policy "to expedite the operation." To this end, Ladimer told Shannon that the proposal for the Normals program was to go from Rourke to General Counsel Banta for submission to the surgeon general and then to the cabinet level: "I believe that the Secretary's Office will want to review this program since it is a new policy with public relations implications."

55. Memo "Not for general release. Volunteers participation in research studies at the Clinical Center, National Institutes of Health," February 15, 1954, PRPL, NIH.

56. Transcript of quarterly clinical staff meeting, January 9, 1958, LOC INTRA 2-1-A, p. 20, ODEF, NIH.

57. *NIH Record*, June 21, 1960. Folder: National Institutes of Health, 1954, MCA correspondence, IX-6-3, MCA.

58. The 1966–67 Annual Report summarized, "Volunteers are older and more mature than other college students we have had to use in the past. This has resulted in a healthier group of student volunteers who are more dedicated to educational and service goals rather than those more interested in civil disobedience." The 1967–68 Annual Report said, "The maturity and motivational aspects of this year's volunteer group has continued to improve with only a few minor exceptions. These exceptions are usually young men who show a greater than ever resistance to being clean shaven and well barbered. Also the mode of dress for our female volunteers appears to have changed where they favor the wearing of shorts and jeans to an ever greater degree than in the past. By this token they resist the policies of the Clinical Center for more appropriate dress." PRPL, NIH.

59. Minutes of Clinical Center Department and section head meeting, September 7, 1971, box 3, folder 6, RG 443/CC, NARAII. Director Nye gives an overview of the Normals program and demographics of its subjects. Of interest to scholars of gender, science, and knowledge production, women who were on the contraceptive pill

could not come to the Clinical Center as part of the Normals program because of the possibility of drug interactions.

60. Hardy to Kliewer, August 2, 1954, folder: National Institutes of Health, 1954, MCA correspondence, IX-6-3, MCA.

61. Zimmerman record, MRD, NIH.

62. Topping, *Recollections*, 126. Another reason for the campaign was that the Clinical Center rubbed local doctors the wrong way. Medical Board meeting minutes, October 27, 1953, box 1, folder Minutes, January 6, 1953–May 1954, Med Board, NIH.

63. I thank Robert Martensen for framing this as an issue of *patronage*, a term that suggests historical continuities in debates over knowledge and money.

64. Although the 1947 Steelman Report, commissioned by the Harry Truman administration, stressed the importance of medical research above all other scientific priorities, funding for NIH did not reach epic proportions until 1956. Nonetheless, in the wake of World War II, NIH leaders got wartime research contracts formerly administered by the Office of Scientific Research and Development transferred to NIH, which not only brought more funding to NIH, but also gave NIH the privilege of sponsoring extramural studies, previously allowed only for the National Cancer Institute. For the importance of the contracts-to-grants maneuver for the subsequent growth of NIH's extramural program, see Fox, "NIH Extramural Program." For a retelling of the meeting in which NIH director Dyer accepted the bounty of contracts that the army and the navy had declined, see Strickland, *Politics, Science, and Dread Disease*, chap. 2. The extramural program already in place within the NIH's National Cancer Institute was on a small scale. Mullan, *Plagues and Politics*. For participants' reflections, see Allen, "NIH Grant Research."

65. Most notably, Surgeon General Thomas Parran had been a personal friend (and appointee) of Franklin Roosevelt, an outspoken New Dealer committed to state-based health care, and an overt populist Democrat with an activist style. Truman removed Parran as head of the Public Health Service in 1948, and the subsequent surgeon general, Leonard Scheele, credited his overt lack of political involvement for his own seven-year endurance in the post. Mullan, *Plagues and Politics*.

66. Creager, "Mobilizing Biomedicine," 189; Greenberg, *Politics of Pure Science*; Lyons, *70 Acres of Science*.

67. The NIH director told the Clinical Center's Medical Board in 1954 that the intramural clinical research program was "not entirely accepted and our program is watched very closely. To a great extent, this is due to the fact that we are a government medical group. One way in which we might help this situation is by more use of our consultants who represent the top people in medicine." Remarks by the director, September 28, 1954, box 1, folder 2, Med Board, NIH. On the seductions of industry and Topping's subsequent post at the University of Pennsylvania, see Topping, *Recollections*. On the unusual hiring practices of NIH, see Park, "Intramural Research Program"; Rossiter, *Women Scientists in America*. It is worth noting that a woman, Oveta Culp Hobby, was the first secretary of the Department of Health, Education, and Welfare, although she had to step down because of a vaccine research scandal in 1955. The ostensible reason for her leaving the post was her husband's ill health. Hobby was in a remarkable position of both power and vulnerability, unusual for the time. She deserves her own biography.

68. The minutes of a 1954 meeting record that a church representative "asked if more than one Institute or project uses one volunteer" and continued, "Mr Ladimer said yes." Meeting minutes, April 12, 1954, PRPL, NIH. In addition, the discussions re-

corded in the Medical Board meeting minutes took for granted that Normals were passed between institutes. E.g., Medical Board meeting minutes, October 9, 1956, box 1, folder "Minutes, Jan 10 1956–Dec 11 1956," Med Board, NIH. My count of Carl's studies is from Zimmerman record, MRD, NIH.

69. Medical Board meeting minutes, September 23, 1952, box 1, "Minutes of Meetings, Med Bd, 1952–69," folder 3, RG 443/CC, NARAII (entries 41–43 in A1; finding aid: 443:130:69:28:01–03). The Medical Board meeting minutes in ACC 0791 at NLM, NIH, start in 1953. For earlier meeting minutes of the same group, see RG 443/CC, NARAII.

70. In a memo, Topping suggested Wilder as task force leader and reminded institute directors that as of 1951 there had already been discussions about "policies of the NIH having to do with studies and investigations on human subjects." Topping also told directors they would bat around proposals at the November 22, 1951, meeting. Topping's memo originally appointed Charles Kidd, a lawyer, as executive secretary, but that appeared to fall through, and Ladimer filled the role. Topping, associate director of NIH, to all institute directors, October 19, 1951, file LOC INTRA 2-1-A, ODEF, NIH. See also Glantz, "Influence of the Nuremberg Code."

71. For the first mention of what later became the Wilder Committee, see Topping, associate director of NIH, to all institute directors, October 19, 1951, file LOC INTRA 2-1-A, ODEF, NIH. On the centrality of softball to the NIH community circa 1950, see "Batter Up! April 10 (Weather Permitting)" *NIH Record*, March 27, 1950; Topping, *Recollections*.

72. For contemporary understandings of the power dynamics of this group, see January 9, 1952, box 1, folder 3, RG 443/CC, NARAII. Appendix A, Minutes of Meeting, Medical Board, March 2, 1953: "In brief, it is the responsibility of the Medical Board to set and preserve high standards of medical care and ethics, to serve as a guiding board for the Director of the Clinical Center, and to recommend medical care policy to the Director of NIH."

73. Confidential administrative memo, July 1, 1957, file LOC INTRA 2-1-A, ODEF, NIH. This memo also says that the group-consideration guidelines were developed by the "Wilder Committee" that existed in 1952, with Ladimer as executive secretary and Wilder as chairman.

74. Minutes of Ad Hoc Committee, December 1964, box 5, folder 1, RG 443/CC, NARAII. Mider was asked to give a history of the group-consideration guidelines to a committee reviewing the document ten years after its creation.

75. On the work of Dr. Andrew Ivy, who had a central role in the American prosecution of Nazi doctors and did contemporaneous research on U.S. prisoners, see Comfort, "Prisoner as Model Organism." For an enlightening story of the relationship between the American Medical Association (AMA) Code of Ethics and the Nuremberg Code, see Weindling, "Origins of Informed Consent."

76. The Department of Defense correspondence was not declassified until the 1990s. *Final Report*, ACHRE, NARAII.

77. "Dress Code Reminder." For a record of interactions and correspondence between NIH researchers and other defense scientists, see the contents of box S09F01B0087, Series: Research Collections, Advisory Committee on Human Radiation Experiments, RG 220, NARAII.

78. Transcript of quarterly clinical staff meeting, January 9, 1958, LOC INTRA 2-1-A, p. 16, ODEF, NIH. This was point five of the ten commandments of medical research involving human subjects as explained to the Clinical Center staff by Dr. Kenneth

Chapman. The Nuremberg Code is widely considered to have had little effect in U.S. law. Glantz, "Influence of the Nuremberg Code"; Katz, *Silent World*; Moreno, "Reassessing the Influence."

79. Harkness, *Research behind Bars*, 152. Harkness writes that Americans felt that the Nuremberg Code applied "only to truly evil scientists." Leading NIH researchers, such as Michael Shimkin, embodied the tension of an upstanding researcher working to improve medical ethics while making questionable choices in his own work. See Shimkin, "Scientific Investigations on Man."

80. Ladimer, "Human Experimentation." Ladimer published his talk in the *New England Journal of Medicine* in 1957. The article shows that Ladimer was aware of the Nuremberg Code and that he fitted human subjects into an animal model of research protection.

81. Informal report, "Coversations [*sic*] at National Institutes of Health," memo by A. Stauffer Curry, box MCA correspondence IX-6-3, folder "National Institutes of Health, 1954," MCA.

82. Shapin, *Scientific Life*.

83. Mandel, "Beacon of Hope." See also Medical Board meeting minutes, October 9, 1956, box 1, folder "Minutes of the Medical Board, Jan 10 1956–Dec 11 1956," Med Board, NIH. A Normal typically "actually participates in more than one institute," so the Medical Board decided to use the signature of the Clinical Center director on certificates, not the signature of a representative of the institute.

84. Medical Board meeting minutes, July 14, 1953, box 1, folder 3, RG 443/CC, NARAII.

85. Medical Board meeting minutes, November 25, 1952, box 1, folder 3, "Minutes of the Medical Board, 1952–54," RG 443/CC, NARAII. Under the heading of "Consent Forms," the minutes of this meeting record that NIH director Trautman "stated that Mr. Rourke, the attorney for the Clinical Center, is interested in the thinking of the various Institutes with regard to 'consent' or 'release' forms which will be signed by patients upon entering a particular project. Mr. Rourke will be invited to attend the next meeting of the Board at which time this subject will be discussed." Rourke did not persuade clinicians in the subsequent meetings.

86. On behalf of Shannon, who had planned to attend the Wilder Committee meeting, Ladimer said, "National Institutes of Health contemplated a local committee on clinical investigation probably to be attached to the Clinical Center Medical Board. This local committee would consider specific problems relating to research projects." The committee described came to be known as the Clinical Research Committee of the Medical Board. In the meeting, they agreed that the Wilder Committee's goal was "to consider those aspects of clinical research involving unestablished procedures in diagnosis and therapy and use of volunteers, healthy and ill, subject to risk." See Meeting minutes of Committee on Principles Governing Clinical Research, January 19, 1953; summary meeting, December 23, 1952, both in INTRA 2-1-A, ODEF, NIH. This summary explains that the purpose of the Wilder Committee would be to develop "a set of principles which may be used as a guide in the formulation and conduct of specific research projects," which would serve as "internal policy." The policy would set "criteria" for, among other things, "reviewing and approving proposals for research involving human subjects." In addition, NIH director Trautman told the Medical Board, "The question was raised also as to the possibility of the Board's interest in clinical investigation where hazard to the individual might be involved, and as to whether or not the Board should assume some responsibility regarding policy

in this regard. Dr. Brown presented for discussion a draft on this subject; i.e., 'The Committee on Clinical Investigation shall be consulted by any investigator prior to the undertaking of any experimental procedure involving any degree of hazard to a patient except when the procedure or medication in question is accepted for the purpose and commonly used by physicians in the routine care of patients. This committee will advise the Medical Policy Committee as to the advisability of undertaking the investigation in question and the Medical Policy Committee will, in turn, advise the Director, NIH, through the Director of the Clinical Center.' It was agreed, however, that this question should not be decided at this time but should be deferred for further consideration pending receipt of information regarding the report to be made by Dr. Wilder to the Institute Directors." Medical Board Meeting Minutes, March 13, 1952, box 1, folder 3, "Meeting minutes, 1952–4," RG 443/CC, NARAII.

87. Report of Clinical Research Committee of the Medical Board, box 1, folder 3, "Meeting minutes, 1952–4," NIH (no date, but probably spring 1953), RG 443/CC, NARAII.

88. For example, Dr. Vernon Knight, clinical director of the National Institute of Allergy and Infectious Disease, maintained in 1965 that "patients with disease who come into the hospital implicitly consent to conventional therapy by virtue of the fact that they have come in voluntarily." Minutes, Ad Hoc Committee, June 11, 1965, box 5, folder 1, RG 443/CC, NARAII. On postwar standards of hazardous research, see also Kutcher, *Contested Medicine*.

89. "Meeting minutes, 1952–4," March 9, 1954, box 1, folder 3, RG 443/CC, NARAII. They required approval of "all projects which required participation of normal volunteers . . . whether or not they are considered hazardous." This was because healthy people, board members felt, "could not be fitted into the normal patient physician relationships." This was the recollection of Mider, as expressed in Minutes of Ad Hoc Committee, December 1964, box 5, folder 1, RG 443/CC, NARAII.

90. Transcript of quarterly clinical staff meeting, January 9, 1958, LOC INTRA 2-1-A, p. 7, ODEF, NIH.

91. Medical Board meeting minutes, June 14, 1960, box 1, folder "Minutes of the medical board April 14 1959–March 28 1961," Med Board, NIH.

92. Medical Board meeting minutes, December 8, 1953, box 1, Med Board, NIH.

93. In an impressive feat of historical analysis, Sydney Halpern demonstrates that epidemiologists in the early twentieth century shared unspoken standards for how to protect human subjects at their local research sites (see Halpern, *Lesser Harms*). Likewise, Jones and Martensen ("Human Radiation Experiments") document how scientists at University of California research facilities discussed the ways in which healthy volunteers (in this case, prisoners) should be treated in clinical settings. The Clinical Center's group-review guidelines were similar in spirit to these earlier efforts. But the Clinical Center guidelines differed in one crucial aspect: they were formally codified federal policy.

94. Medical Board meeting minutes, March 13, 1952, Clinical Center, "Meeting minutes 1952–4," box 1, folder 3, RG 443, NARAII. As of February 1953, the official function of the Medical Board was to develop "policies governing standards of medical care at the Clinical Center." The following month, the board's minutes articulated their mission as "to set and preserve high standards of medical care and ethics." Minutes of meeting, Medical Board, March 2, 1953, ibid.

95. Minutes of Ad Hoc Committee, February 16, April 23, June 11, 1965, box 5, folder 1, RG 443/CC, NARAII.

96. Minutes of meeting, Medical Board, March 2, 1953, box 1, folder 3, RG 443/CC, NARAII.

CHAPTER FIVE

Epigraph: Irving Ladimer, "Safeguards for Drug Testing," paper presented to Schering Corp., November 12, 1964. It was also attached to an undated note to Dr. Henry K. Beecher. Box 11, Subjects, human experimentation; folder 41, Ladimer, Irving 1961–1965, Beecher papers.

1. Isaac chart, p. 9/14, narrative summary, MRD, NIH. The names of all healthy patients in this book are pseudonyms.

2. Novak, "LSD before Leary." LSD was discovered in 1943 and became available in the United States in 1949. It was first thought to be a therapy for mental illnesses such as addiction and schizophrenia. Charles Savage said that in 1949 he started looking, with navy funding, "for improved methods of inducing psychocatharsis and facilitating psychotherapy." He continued: "I ran through the gamut of alkaloids, from mescaline and cannabis, through marmine, marmaline, ascopolamine, and cocaine. I was primarily interested in mescaline, but was dismayed by the intense nausea it produced both in me and in my patients. When I learned from Dr. Beringer that LSD produced 'ein süsser Rausch' [a more pleasant high] than mescaline, I began to use it and have been working with it on and off ever since." He was "impressed" by the similarities between an LSD-induced state and schizophrenia itself. Savage's aim was to understand "the meaning of the LSD experience." Abramson, *Use of LSD in Psychotherapy*, 9. On psychiatric drug programs at the Clinical Center, see Farreras, Hannaway, and Harden, *Mind, Brain, Body, and Behavior.*

   Richard Riseberg, legal adviser, NIH, to Sidney Edelman, assistant general counsel for PHS, Subject: LSD Research, April 7, 1976, box 26, folder Gov Rel 2-10 NIH-CIA MK-ULTRA project, 1976–79, RG 443, NARAII. Edelman asked, via a memo to James Isbister (administrator, Alcohol, Drug Abuse, and Mental Health Administration) on January 9, 1976, that the legal department review LSD research. This report and its supporting documents paint a rich picture of the research on LSD going on at the Clinical Center (and in Lexington) in the 1950s and 1960s—as well as the changing methods for getting informed consent, both for sick patients and Normals (including prisoners). There were sixty projects involving 1,750 human subjects (sick and healthy) in therapeutic and nontherapeutic LSD studies. The Clinical Center got LSD from Sandoz Pharmaceuticals. LSD was categorized as an illicit drug in 1966. The CIA did fund LSD research at the NIMH Intramural Program at Lexington, KY, under Harold Isbell, and the results were published. Subjects did consent, but consent at that time (the report notes) did not require written documentation. For some more skeptical views, see Savage, "LSD-25."

3. Novak, "LSD before Leary." This article describes the early history of LSD and explains that researchers did not start to think of LDS as dangerous until 1960, following the work of Sidney Cohen. Novak mentions Savage's LSD research on Mennonites in note 13. Contemporary accounts suggest that some clinicians were very uneasy about LSD prior to 1960, however. Savage told a group of therapists in 1960, for example, that "perhaps we should spend a little more time on this problem of derogatory attitudes towards LSD. I encountered them, and I believe they had considerable effect on some of the results." From his perspective in 1960, Savage explained that negative attitudes about LSD had "persisted and until 1954 the use of such drugs made one very suspect." Abramson, *Use of LSD in Psychotherapy*, 29. By 1967 the Normals pro-

gram leaders reported that there were fewer volunteers because "many parents were reluctant to sign the voluntary consent forms for their children to join us because of apprehensions over the use of experiment [sic] drugs and the use of radio active [sic] isotopes." Annual Report, 1967–68, PRPL, NIH.

4. Isaac chart, p. 9/14, narrative summary, MRD, NIH.
5. Katz, *Silent World*.
6. Faden and Beauchamp, *History and Theory*.
7. Carpenter, *Reputation and Power*.
8. Shannon himself did use consent forms during World War II. He had trained Berliner at Goldwater Hospital during the war (see chapter 4). As of 1958, it was Clinical Center policy to get signed forms from Normals. Nonetheless, during the autumn of 1960, when Himmelsbach was advocating signed forms, Berliner was the most vocal advocate of having a Normal policy that did not require signed forms, most likely because the prisoner program was starting at the Clinical Center (see chapter 6). Medical Board meeting minutes, October 11, 25; November 8, 1960, box 1, folder Minutes of the Medical Board, April 14, 1959–March 28, 1961, Med Board, NIH.
9. See, for example, Medical Board meeting minutes, October 9, 1956, box 1, folder Minutes of the Medical Board, January 10, 1956–December 11, 1956, Med Board, NIH.
10. Isaac record, MRD, NIH.
11. Medical Board meeting minutes, October 23, 1956, box 1, folder Minutes of the Medical Board, January 10, 1956–December 11, 1956, Med Board, NIH. As of 1957, the content of the medical records was also considered inadequate by the Medical Board. The board members asked for better records of circumstances of patients' deaths, and they also debated whether the opinions of physicians with whom researchers disagreed could be removed from charts. Their decision was "no." Medical Board meeting minutes, July 23, 1957, box 1, folder Minutes of the Medical Board, January 8, 1957–November 26, 1957, Med Board, NIH.
12. Medical Board meeting minutes, June 10, 1958, box 1, folder Minutes of the Medical Board, December 10, 1957–March 24, 1959, Med Board, NIH.
13. Carole Spearin, "CC Medical Record Dept.," *NIH Record*, November 7, 1961, 2.
14. Lipscomb, "Professional Boundaries." The occupation of medical record librarian grew out of medical libraries, places where doctors and students had gone to look at books and journals since about 1910. There were also record clerks, beginning around 1930. There was a movement toward standardizing medical records in hospitals around the 1930s. Because of confusion over the two professions of medical book librarian and medical record librarian, and for professionalization, the two professional organizations tried to sort out the definitions in the 1950s.
15. Garfinkel argues that the act of documenting in hospitals was a form of social control of patients, which is why, he argues, hospital employees fetishized documentation, even though the documents he studied were quite poorly kept. *Studies in Ethnomethodology*. See also chapter 3.
16. Some of it was shoddy recordkeeping. In 1961, for example, four Normals did not sign "project release" forms as they were supposed to. Report of medical record audit, January 6, 1961, PRPL, NIH.
17. McCarthy, "Institutional Review Boards."
18. Faden and Beauchamp, *History and Theory*.
19. "Meeting Minutes, 1952–4," December 2, 1952, box 1, folder 3, RG 443/CC, NARAII.

20. This statement is based on my review of the records of thirty of the earliest Normal controls who came to the Clinical Center through the Mennonite and Brethren service organizations between 1954 and 1958.

21. Memo, "Evidence Substantiating the Requirement That Normal Volunteers Give Signatory Consent to Participate in Research Projects in the Clinical Center," October 18, 1960, attached to February 5, 1965, meeting minutes, box 1, folder October 13, 1964–January 25, 1966, Med Board, NIH.

22. Isaac record, p. 2959, MRD, NIH.

23. Isaac record, MRD, NIH.

24. Faden and Beauchamp, *History and Theory*, 126.

25. Transcript of quarterly clinical staff meeting, January 9, 1958, LOC INTRA 2-1-A, p. 43, ODEF, NIH.

26. Ibid., p. 44.

27. Rothman's classic *Strangers at the Bedside* is perhaps a main source of this interpretation of Beecher. I thank Robert Martensen for helpful conversations about this matter. See William J. Curran and Henry K. Beecher, "Experimentation in Children: A Reexamination of Legal Ethical Principles," *Journal of the American Medical Association* 210, no. 1 (1969): 77–83.

28. Rourke, "Experimentation in Children," 301.

29. Faden and Beauchamp, *History and Theory*, 125–27. Historians have shown that the term *informed consent* was actually used by the Department of Defense a decade earlier, but the documents in which it was used were classified.

30. On doctors' changing conceptions of the sick patients' clarity of mind, particularly as it overlapped with doctors' biases toward different social groups, see Faden and Beauchamp, *History and Theory*. On the structure of professional competition with the medical marketplace and its effects on patient care, see Starr, *Social Transformation of American Medicine*; Katz, *Experimentation with Human Beings*.

31. "Meeting Minutes, 1952–4," December 2, 1952, box 1, folder 3, RG 443/CC, NARAII.

32. Ladimer, "Safeguards for Drug Testing"; Ladimer and Newman, *Clinical Investigation in Medicine*, 140.

33. Ladimer to Beecher, undated (probably November 1964), box 11, H MS c 64, Beecher papers. Ladimer presented the paper on November 12, 1964.

34. Dr. Chapman, Clinical Center, Transcript of quarterly clinical staff meeting, January 9, 1958, p. 18, ODEF, NIH.

35. Ibid.

36. E.g., Lasagna and von Felsinger, "Volunteer Subject in Research."

37. Lasagna did not mention this to Clinical Center researchers, and it may not have entered into his mind, but his findings were based on Normals taking part in LSD studies. Ibid.

38. Isaac record, MRD, NIH.

39. Acting chief, lab of Clinical Science, NIMH, to associate director of CC (Himmelsbach), June 22, 1960, PRPL, NIH.

40. "Annual Report," 1967–68, PRPL, NIH.

41. In the meeting, Cohen cited Pollin and Perlin, "Psychiatric Evaluation."

42. Minutes of Ad Hoc Committee, May 28, 1965, box 5, folder 1, RG 443/CC, NARAII.

43. Minutes of Ad Hoc Committee, June 2, 1965, box 5, folder 1, RG 443/CC, NARAII.

44. Medical Board meeting minutes, October 11, 1960, box 1, folder Minutes of the Medical Board, April 14, 1959–March 28 1961, Med Board, NIH.

45. Memo, "Evidence Substantiating the Requirement That Normal Volunteers Give Sig-

natory Consent to Participate in Research Projects in the Clinical Center," October 18, 1960, attached to February 5, 1965, meeting minutes, box 1, folder October 13, 1964–January 25, 1966, Med Board, NIH.

46. There were extensive discussions throughout the autumn of 1960 over whether researchers "must" or "may" collected signed consent forms, because the prisoner program was beginning. See especially Medical Board meeting minutes, October 11, 25; November 8, 1960, Med Board, NIH.

47. Isaac record, 3002, 31/32, batch 5, MRD, NIH

CHAPTER SIX

1. Maginnis to Himmelsbach, January 6, 1961, "Report," PRPL, NIH. The Medical Board's January 14, 1964, minutes give a specific example of protocol for a malaria study, and the minutes record that "infection would be produced at the NIH, utilizing infected mosquitoes." Folder Medical board meeting minutes, February 12, 1963–September 22, 1964, Med Board, NIH.

2. Smith, "1000th Prisoner Volunteer Admitted."

3. The Bureau of Prisons stated that researchers should get written approval of the institution's research committee and warden, which included written evidence of prior review of the project by institution associates of the investigator who are not directly involved in the research. See Dr. Vernon Knight's discussion of prisoner consent procedures: meeting minutes, folder 1, Ad hoc committee to review certain considerations of clin. res. procedure, June 11, 1965, box 5, minutes of meetings, RG 443/CC, NARAII.

4. Glantz, "Influence of the Nuremberg Code"; Harkness, "Significance of the Nuremberg Code."

5. For an excellent case study that complicates boundaries between research and subjects, as well as conventional notions of consent, see Comfort, "Prisoner as Model Organism."

6. Knight, "Volunteers in Medical Virology"; Lederer, "Research without Borders," 208.

7. 1965–66 Annual Report, submitted by Delbert Nye, PRPL, NIH.

8. Annual Report, 1964–65 (July 1–June 30), PRPL, NIH. This report states that there were 639 volunteers (an increase of 57 from 582 the previous year). There had been a National Institute of Allergy and Infectious Disease Prisoner Volunteer Program, which brought in "24 new virus volunteers every 5 weeks." Twelve institutions sent prisoners.

9. Himmelsbach was appointed associate director of the Clinical Center in the autumn of 1959. Medical Board meeting minutes, October 27, 1959, box 1, folder Minutes of the Medical Board, April 14, 1959–March 28, 1961, Med Board, NIH. Also see Oral History with Clifton Himmelsbach, November 2, 1994, Substance Abuse Research Center, University of Michigan, http://sitemaker.umich.edu/substance.abuse .history/home.

10. Carpenter. *Reputation and Power*; Ladimer, "Human Experimentation." On the consequences of the FDA drug amendments, see Lasagna, "New Drug Development." Himmelsbach was appointed associate director of the Clinical Center in the autumn of 1959. Medical Board meeting minutes, October 27, 1959, box 1, folder Minutes of the Medical Board, April 14, 1959–March 28, 1961, Med Board, NIH. Also see Oral History with Clifton Himmelsbach and Jon Harkness and researchers through the University of Michigan: http://sitemaker.umich.edu/substance.abuse.history/ oral_history_interviews&mode=single&recordID=2487230&nextMode=list.

11. Campbell, Olsen, and Walden, *Narcotic Farm*; Campbell, *Discovering Addiction*.

12. Oral History with Clifton Himmelsbach, November 2, 1994, Substance Abuse Research Center, University of Michigan, http://sitemaker.umich.edu/substance.abuse .history/home.
13. Annual Report, 1964–65, 1965–66, NVPP, PRPL, NIH.
14. Smith, "1000th Prisoner Volunteer Admitted."
15. Annual Reports of the Normal Volunteer Patient Program, Building 61, upstairs filing cabinet, PRPL, NIH. No annual reports are available for the prisoner program in 1966–67 and 1967–68. I thank Lauren Feld for creating a chart from the Normal Volunteer Patient Program annual reports (see chapter 4, note 3).
16. Annual Reports, 1964–65, 1965–66, PRPL, NIH.
17. Mandel, "Beacon of Hope"; "Dr. Jack Masur."
18. Mandel, "Beacon of Hope"; "Dr. Jack Masur."
19. February 11, 1964, minutes, box 1, Med Board, NIH. The article was written by Elinor Langer and published on February 7, 1964.
20. Langer, "Human Experimentation"; Katz, *Experimentation with Human Beings.*
21. The suit was known informally within NIH as the Southam case, after the PHS-funded primary investigator, Chester Southam. "Ad Hoc Committee," Minutes of meeting, February 24, 1966, box 5, folder 1, RG 443, NARAII; Curran, "Government Regulation of Use of Human Subjects."
22. Katz, *Experimentation with Human Beings*, 64.
23. The NIH budget steadily increased from $98 million to $294 million over those three years. See Shannon, "National Institutes of Health: Critical Years," table 2.
24. Shannon, "National Institutes of Health: Problems," 178. Starr, *Social Transformation of American Medicine*; Strickland, *Politics, Science, and Dread Disease.*
25. Shannon, "National Institutes of Health: Critical Years." On drinking habits, see Strickland, *Politics, Science, and Dread Disease*, 186.
26. Strickland, *Politics, Science, and Dread Disease*, 101. Strickland also writes that by the early 1960s, "the Surgeon General of the Public Health Service was a decreasingly important figure. So was the Secretary of Health, Education, and Welfare, except when periodically called upon to arbitrate major or minor disputes" (132).
27. This phrase in particular is attributed to Congressman Laird (R-WI). Ibid., 115.
28. The charge against NIH was led by Lawrence H. Fountain (D-NC), chairman of the Intergovernmental Relations Subcommittee of the House Government Operations Committee. Tellingly, Ernest Allen, one of the first staffers of NIH's Office of Research Grants, wrote that of the many "grant procedures and policies developed in the early years of [the extramural] program," it was "scientific freedom of the principal investigator, [that stood as] perhaps the most important single concept." Allen, "NIH Research Grants," 3.
29. Shannon did not argue that NIH investigators were good money managers; rather, he asserted that the loose budget management was by design: "This grant of freedom to the investigator is deliberate and in response to a fundamental philosophy. It is not a consequence of inability to place tight controls over the expenditure of funds. The basic component of this philosophy is that science will advance more rapidly, and that as a consequence, practical findings will emerge most rapidly and in the greatest profusion, if science is unfettered by restrictions—if scientists are given freedom to follow their ideas." Shannon's associate director for research grants, Ernest Allen, drew the line most tightly between good science and what the Fountain Committee regarded as bad management when he argued that "scientific freedom calls for considerable budget freedom." *Hearings before a Subcommittee of the Committee*

on Governmental Operations," Committee on Governmental Operations, 87th Cong., 2nd sess., 1962, pp. 14, 24. Such comments left the impression that NIH leaders were "operating in never-never land," "romanticiz[ing] research," and suggested that an investigator would need to "figure in the time that he uses for meditation," in the words of Delphis Goldberg, Fountain's staff aide in the investigation. Greenberg, "NIH and Fountain," 1077.

30. Shannon was reportedly furious with his staff for not warning him that his testimony would be taken extremely seriously, which suggests that this was one of the few moments out of the many that Shannon spent testifying before Congress in which he had his guard down. See Strickland, *Politics, Science, and Dread Disease,* chap. 7.

31. A supporter of Shannon caustically claimed that this was Fountain's favorite phrase to "quote and criticize" but acknowledged that "'trivial' was the wrong word." Dael Wolfle, "Achievement and Management," *Science* 158 (1967): 721. Strickland's read of this utterance is that Shannon "f[ell] back on that cliché-conviction dear to the hearts of established, well-funded scientists" and in doing so "committed what is perhaps the cardinal sin of legislative-executive etiquette. . . . Shannon suggested to the committee that it was pursuing a minor theme, or worse." Strickland, *Politics, Science, and Dread Disease,* 174.

32. Greenberg, "NIH and Fountain."

33. Shannon to Rep. Fulton, April 20, 1964, box 1, folder "DRG 1962–1968," 557, NLM, NIH. Shannon quoted the Fountain Committee on investigators' "moral obligations" and wrote, "[I] regret the necessity for activities which distract scientists from concentrating on their research"; he hoped that institutions would be able to implement the new rules in a way that would "preserve the scientific or professional freedom of the research personnel."

34. Several scathing investigator responses to the Fountain Committee reforms were kept in the files of the NIH Office of the Director, box 1, 557, NLM, NIH; e.g., Arnold Welch, "The New Regulations Pertaining to Research Grants of the Public Health Service," *Science* 141 (1963): 1099–1100, 1102, 1104. Also see the contents of box 32, folder "Regulations," General Correspondence, RG 443/DRG, NARAII.

35. "Biomedical Science and Its Administration: A Study of the National Institutes of Health," 1965, Washington, DC, 18. Shannon's copy of the report is in box 22, 363, NLM, NIH. Good summaries of the report and outlines of how the committee itself worked include Joseph Cooper, "Onward the Management of Science: The Wooldridge Report," *Science* 148 (1965): 1433–39; Philip H. Abelson, "Biomedical Science and Its Administration," *Science* 148 (1965): 171. The Wooldridge Report did endorse (without explicit mention) many of the suggestions made by the Fountain Committee, such as greater decentralization of grant administration into universities for better accountability.

36. Greenberg, "NIH and Fountain," 1076.

37. See William Curran's forward to Ladimer and Newman, *Clinical Investigation in Medicine.*

38. According to its director, William Curran, the Law-Medicine Research Institute replicated a 1961 study by Louis Welt, who used the phrase "committee of disinterested faculty." Curran, "Government Regulation."

39. Ladimer's data are available in several places. I used a paper that Ladimer sent to Henry Beecher shortly after his results came in. "Survey of Professional Journals: Editorial Responsibility in Clinical Research," attached to Ladimer to Beecher, October 30, 1961, box 11, Beecher papers.

40. Livingston's official title was associate chief for program development, Division of Facilities and Resources, NIH. The best overview of this episode, and the most complete publication of its primary sources that I have seen, is Frankel, "Human Experimentation in the United States." A description of the committee (including members) from within NIH is in box 5, "Minutes of Meetings," folder 1, "Ad Hoc Committee," Minutes of meeting, December 30, 1964, RG 443, NARAII.

41. Quoted in Curran, "Government Regulation of Use of Human Subjects." Much has been made of Shannon's letter to Surgeon General Terry in 1965 stating that a high priority should be given to formulating these principles. Shannon wrote there that "a broader approach" than the professional group suggested by Livingston "may be necessary," such that the group "includes representatives of the whole ethical, moral, and legal interests of society." Shannon's letter to Terry is described to this effect in Curran, "Government Regulation of Use of Human Subjects"; and in Robert Veatch, "Human Experimentation Committees: Professional or Representative?" *Hastings Center Report* 5 (1975): 31–40.

42. Memo from assistant chief, Division of Hospitals (Robert Lashmutt), "Subject: Attendance at National Advisory Health Council Meeting, Sept 28, 1965," October 1, 1965, folder 2, Ethical, Moral and Legal Aspects, CC, ONIHH, NIH.

43. Carpenter, *Reputation and Power*; Tobbell, "Allied against Reform"; Curran, "Government Regulation of Use of Human Subjects."

44. Javits to Terry, Terry to Javits, both June 15, 1965, folder 2, Ethical, Moral and Legal Aspects, CC, ONIHH, NIH.

45. Terry to Javits, June 15, 1965, folder 2, Ethical, Moral and Legal Aspects, CC, ONIHH, NIH. With seeming indignation, Terry continued that informed consent was "an extension of a long standing tradition and legal requirement" and that "the circumstances of the physician-patient relationship [had] always required obtaining the consent of the patient."

46. Masur to Javits, September 13, 1965, folder 2, Ethical, Moral and Legal Aspects, CC, ONIHH, NIH.

47. Willcox to Dempsey, July 13, 1965, folder 2, Ethical, Moral and Legal Aspects, CC, ONIHH, NIH.

48. Terry to Javits, July 1965, folder 2, Ethical, Moral and Legal Aspects, CC, ONIHH, NIH. Willcox to Dempsey, July 13, 1965, folder 2, Ethical, Moral and Legal Aspects, CC, ONIHH, NIH. Willcox quotes Rourke directly. It appears that Terry did not get this feedback soon enough to incorporate it into a fresh draft to Javits.

49. *Final Report*, ACHRE, RG 220, NARAII.

50. Rourke to Terry, September 16, 1965, folder 2, Ethical, Moral and Legal Aspects, CC, ONIHH, NIH.

51. Rourke to Stewart, October 26, 1965, folder 2, Ethical, Moral and Legal Aspects, CC, ONIHH, NIH.

52. National Advisory Health Council, agenda, September 27–28, 1965, folder 2, Ethical, Moral and Legal Aspects, CC, ONIHH, NIH.

53. "Proposal for discussion," September 28, 1965, p. 2, folder 2, Ethical, Moral and Legal Aspects, CC, ONIHH, NIH. The draft resolution from Shannon's office states that because of experimental methods in which patient therapy may conflict with knowledge production, "the judgmental exclusiveness of the physician-patient relationship is inadequate."

54. Memo from Joseph Murtaugh, November 2, 1965; memo from Reisman to Masur, December 6, 1965, both in folder 2, Ethical, Moral and Legal Aspects, CC, ONIHH, NIH.

55. Memo to the Heads of Institutions Conducting Research with Public Health Service Grants from the Surgeon General, February 8, 1966, folder 2, Ethical, Moral and Legal Aspects, CC, ONIHH, NIH.
56. Ibid.
57. Memo to the Heads of Institutions Receiving Public Health Service Grants from the Surgeon General, July 1, 1966, Policy and Procedure Order 129, folder 2, Ethical, Moral and Legal Aspects, CC, ONIHH, NIH.
58. The use of the phrase "clinical research and investigation" in Stewart's memo title made it unclear whether the policy applied to clinical research as well as all investigations, or to clinical research and clinical investigations. Stewart clarified that he meant the former. Stark, "IRBs in Myth and Practice"; Stark, "Science of Ethics." See also Schrag, *Ethical Imperialism.*
59. Rourke was explaining his view to the surgeon general. Rourke to Stewart, October 26, 1965, folder 2, Ethical, Moral and Legal Aspects, CC, ONIHH, NIH.
60. Carpenter, *Reputation and Power*, 546–72.
61. Curran, "Government Regulation of Use of Human Subjects." On prisoner research in this period, the foundational text is Harkness, *Research behind Bars.*
62. Fletcher, "Location of the Office"; McCarthy, "Reflections on Organizational Locus."
63. McCarthy, "Reflections on Organizational Locus," 230.

CONCLUSION

1. Beecher, "Experimentation in Man"; *Final Report*, 157–59, 177–78, ACHRE, RG 220, NARAII.
2. Beecher, "Ethics and Clinical Research." For an analysis of how Beecher wrote the paper, see Freidenfelds, "Recruiting Allies for Reform."
3. Halpern, "Medical Authority"; Reverby, *Examining Tuskegee*; Skrentny, *Minority Rights Revolution.*
4. Beecher's institution, Massachusetts General Hospital, had anticipated the policy and asked Beecher to take charge of the ethics committee. He begrudgingly accepted and remained opposed to federal oversight of what he felt was a professional duty. See the contents of box 8, Beecher papers.
5. For discussion of the surgeon general's policy, see Meader to Coulter, May 3, 1966, box 8, folder 54, "Committee on Research, Subcommittee on Human Studies: 1965–1967 with Ralph G. Meader," Beecher papers. Beecher was the chair of the Massachusetts General Hospital human-subjects review committee starting in November 1965.
6. Rothman, *Strangers at the Bedside*; Jonsen, *Birth of Bioethics.*
7. I am grateful to John Evans, Ben Hurlbut, and Robert Martensen for countless conversations that have helped me to articulate this point.
8. Bosk, "Professional Ethicist Available"; Cooter, "Resistible Rise of Medical Ethics"; Evans, "History and Future of Bioethics"; Martensen, "History of Bioethics"; Toulmin, "How Medicine Saved the Life of Bioethics."

BIBLIOGRAPHY

MANUSCRIPT COLLECTIONS

American Anthropological Association (AAA). National Anthropology Archives, Smithsonian Institution Support Center, Suitland, MD.

Beecher, Henry K. Papers (H MS c 64). Harvard Medical Library in the Francis A. Countway Library of Medicine, Boston, MA.

Mennonite Church USA Archives (MCA). Goshen, IN

National Academy of Sciences Archive (NAS). Washington, DC.

National Archives and Research Administration II (NARAII). College Park, MD.

   RG 220, Advisory Committee for Human Radiation Experiments (ACHRE), Records of Temporary Committees, Commissions, and Boards

   RG 235, General Records of the Department of Health, Education, and Welfare

   RG 443, Records of the NIH Clinical Center, National Institutes of Health (NIH)

National Institutes of Health (NIH). Bethesda, MD.

   Medical Records Department, Clinical Center, Building 10 (MRD)

   National Library of Medicine (NLM)

   · MS C 363, James A. Shannon Papers.
   · MS C 536, NIH Directors' Files.
   · ACC 0791, NIH Clinical Center Office of Medical Services, 1953–87 (Med Board)

   Office of NIH History, William H. Nacher Building (ONIHH)

   Office of Patient Recruitment and Public Liaison, Building 61 (PRPL)

   Office of the Director Electronic Files, Dr. James A. Shannon Building (ODEF). Maintained and searched by Dr. Richard Mandel.

PUBLISHED SOURCES

Abadie, Roberto. *The Professional Guinea Pig: Big Pharma and the Risky World of Human Subjects*. Durham, NC: Duke University Press, 2010.

Abbott, Lura, and Christine Grady. "A Systematic Review of the Empirical Literature Evaluating IRBs: What We Know and What We Still Need to Learn." *Journal of Empirical Research on Human Research Ethics* 6, no. 1 (2011): 3–20.

Abramson, Harold Alexander. *The Use of LSD in Psychotherapy: Transactions*. New York: Josiah Macy, 1960.

Albala, Ilene, Margaret Doyle, and Paul S. Appelbaum. "The Evolution of Consent Forms for Research: A Quarter Century of Changes." *IRB* 32 no. 3 (2010): 7–11.

Alder, Ken. *The Lie Detectors: The History of an American Obsession*. New York: Free Press, 2007.

Alford, R. H., J. A. Kasel, J. R. Lehrich, and V. Knight. "Human Responses to Experimental Infection with Influenza a/Equi 2 Virus." *American Journal of Epidemiology* 86, no. 1 (1967): 185–92.

Allen, Ernest. "Early Years of NIH Research Grants." NIH Center for Scientific Review, www.cms.csr.nih.gov.

Amadae, Sonja Michelle. *Rationalizing Capitalist Democracy: The Cold War Origins of Rational Choice Liberalism*. Chicago: University of Chicago Press, 2003.

Annas, George J., and Michael A. Grodin, eds. *The Nazi Doctors and the Nuremberg Code*. New York: Oxford University Press, 1992.

Austin, J. L. *How to Do Things with Words*. The William James Lectures. Oxford: Clarendon Press, 1962.

Beauchamp, Tom L., and James F. Childress. *Principles of Biomedical Ethics*. 6th ed. New York: Oxford University Press, 2009.

Beecher, Henry K. "Ethics and Clinical Research." *New England Journal of Medicine* 274, no. 24, 1966: 1354–60.

———. "Experimentation in Man." *Journal of the American Medical Association* 169, no. 5 (1959): 461–78.

Bell, James, John Whiton, and Sharon Connelly. "Final Report: Evaluation of NIH Implementation of Section 491 of the Public Health Service Act, Mandating a Program of Protection for Research Subjects," 1998, James Bell Associates, Arlington, VA.

Bernstein, Basil B. *Class, Codes, and Control: Theoretical Studies towards a Sociology of Language*. New York: Schocken Books, 1975.

Bledsoe, Caroline H., Bruce Sherin, Adam G. Galinsky, Nathalia M. Headley, Carol A. Heimer, Erik Kjeldgaard, James Lindgren, Jon D. Miller, Michael E. Roloff, and David H. Uttal. "Regulating Creativity: Research and Survival in the IRB Iron Cage." *Northwestern University Law Review* 101, no. 2 (2007): 593–642.

Boltanski, Luc, and Laurent Thévenot. *On Justification: Economies of Worth*. Trans. Catherine Porter. Princeton, NJ: Princeton University Press, 2006.

Bosk, Charles L. "Professional Ethicist Available: Logical, Secular, Friendly." *Daedalus* 128, no. 4 (1999): 47–68.

———. *What Would You Do? Juggling Bioethics and Ethnography*. Chicago: University of Chicago Press, 2008.

Bosk, Charles L., and Raymond De Vries. "Bureaucracies of Mass Deception: Institutional Review Boards and the Ethics of Ethnographic Research." In *Annals of the American Academy of Political and Social Sciences* 595, no. 1 (2004): 249–63.

Bosk, Charles L., and Brian Frader. "Institutional Ethics Committees: Sociological Oxymoron, Empirical Black Box." In *Bioethics and Society: Constructing the Ethical Enterprise*, edited by Raymond DeVries and Janardan Subedi, 94–116. New York: Prentice Hall, 1998.

Brandt, Allan. *The Cigarette Century: The Rise, Fall, and Deadly Persistence of the Product That Defined America*. New York: Basic Books, 2007.

———. "Racism and Research: The Case of the Tuskegee Syphilis Study." *Hastings Center Report* 8, no. 6 (1978): 21–29.

Brenneis, Donald. "Discourse and Discipline at the National Research Council: A Bureaucratic Bildungsroman." *Cultural Anthropology* 9, no. 1 (1994): 23–36.

———. "Documenting Ethics." In *Embedding Ethics*, edited by Lynn Meskell and Peter Pels, 239–51. New York: Wenner-Gren, 2005.

———. "Documenting Ethics." Unpublished manuscript, 2002, Santa Cruz, CA.

Brown, Mark B. "Fairly Balanced: The Politics of Representation on Government Advisory Committees." *Political Research Quarterly* 61, no. 4 (2008): 547–60.

Burman, William, Peter Breese, Stephen Weis, Naomi Bock, John Bernardo, and Andrew Vernon. "The Effects of Local Review on Informed Consent Documents from a Multicenter Clinical Trials Consortium." *Controlled Clinical Trials* 24, no. 3 (2003): 245–55.

Cambrosio, Alberto, Peter Keating, Thomas Schlich, and George Weisz. "Regulatory Objectivity and the Generation and Management of Evidence in Medicine." *Social Science and Medicine* 63, no. 1 (2006): 189–99.

Campbell, Nancy. *Discovering Addiction: The Science and Politics of Substance Abuse Research.* Ann Arbor: University of Michigan Press, 2007.

Campbell, Nancy D., J. P. Olsen, and Luke Walden. *The Narcotic Farm: The Rise and Fall of America's First Prison for Drug Addicts.* New York: Harry N. Abrams, 2008.

Carpenter, Daniel P. *Reputation and Power: Organizational Image and Pharmaceutical Regulation at the FDA.* Princeton Studies in American Politics. Princeton, NJ: Princeton University Press, 2010.

Carson, John. *The Measure of Merit: Talents, Intelligence, and Inequality in the French and American Republics, 1750–1940.* Princeton, NJ: Princeton University Press, 2007.

Caute, David. *The Great Fear: The Anti-Communist Purge under Truman and Eisenhower.* London: Secker and Warburg, 1978.

Centeno, Miguel Angel. "The New Leviathan: The Dynamics and Limits of Technocracy." *Theory and Society* 22, no. 3 (1993): 307–35.

Cerulo, Karen A. *Never Saw It Coming: Cultural Challenges to Envisioning the Worst.* Chicago: University of Chicago Press, 2006.

Collins, Harry, and Robert Evans. *Rethinking Expertise.* Chicago: University of Chicago Press, 2007.

Comfort, Nathaniel. "The Prisoner as Model Organism: Malaria Research at Stateville Penitentiary." *Studies in History and Philosophy of Science, Part C,* 40, no. 3 (2009): 190–203.

Cooter, R. "The Resistible Rise of Medical Ethics," *Social History of Medicine* 8, no. 2 (1995): 257–70.

Creager, Angela. "Mobilizing Biomedicine: Virus Research between Lay Health Organizations and the U.S. Federal Government, 1935–1955." In *Biomedicine in the Twentieth Century: Practices, Policies, and Politics,* edited by Caroline Hannaway, 171–201. Amsterdam: IOS Press, 2008.

———. "Molecular Surveillance: A History of the Radioimmunoassays." In *Crafting Immunity: Working Histories of Clinical Immunology,* edited by Kenton Kroker, Pauline M. H. Mazumdar, and Jennifer E. Keelan, 201–30. Aldershot, England: Ashgate, 2008.

———. "Nuclear Energy in the Service of Biomedicine: The US Atomic Energy Commission's Radioisotope Program, 1946–1950." *Journal of the History of Biology* 39, no. 4 (2006): 649–84.

Curran, William J. "Government Regulation of the Use of Human Subjects in Medical Research: The Approach of Two Federal Agencies." *Daedalus* 98, no. 2 (1969): 542–94.

Daston, Lorraine, and Peter Galison. *Objectivity.* New York: Zone Books, 2007.

Dehue, Trudy. "History of the Control Group." In *Encyclopedia of Statistics in Behavioral Science,* edited by Brian Everitt and David Howell, 829–36. Hoboken, NJ: Wiley, 2005.

De Vries, Raymond G., and Carl P. Forsberg. "What Do IRBs Look Like? What Kind of Support Do They Receive?" *Accountability in Research* 9, nos. 3–4 (2002): 199–216.

Dingwall, Robert. "Turn Off the Oxygen." *Law and Society Review* 41, no. 4 (2007): 787–96.

"Dr. Jack Masur, Clinical Center Director, Program Dies Suddenly; Joined PHS in 1943." *NIH Record*, March 18, 1969.

"Sartorial Note." *NIH Record*, October 1, 1951.

Dresser, Rebecca. "First-in-Human Trial Participants: Not a Vulnerable Population, but Vulnerable Nonetheless." *Journal of Law, Medicine, and Ethics* 37, no 1 (2009): 38–50.

Durant, Darrin. "Accounting for Expertise: Wynne and the Autonomy of the Lay Public Actor." *Public Understanding of Science* 17, no. 9 (2008): 5–20.

Eliasoph, Nina, and Paul Lichterman. "Culture in Interaction." *American Journal of Sociology* 108, no. 4 (2003): 735–94.

Elliott, Carl. "Guinea-Pigging." *New Yorker*, January 7, 2008.

Elliott, Carl, and Roberto Abadie. "Exploiting a Research Underclass in Phase 1 Clinical Trials. *New England Journal of Medicine* 358 (2008): 2316–17.

Emanuel, Ezekiel. "Unequal Treatment," review of *Medical Apartheid*, by Harriet A. Washington. *New York Times*, February 18, 2007, Sunday Book Review.

Emanuel, Ezekiel J., Trudo Lemmens, and Carl Elliot. "Should Society Allow Research Ethics Boards to Be Run as For-Profit Enterprises?" *PLoS Medicine* 3, no. 7 (2006): e309.

Epstein, Steven. *Impure Science: AIDS, Activism, and the Politics of Knowledge*. Los Angeles: University of California Press, 1996.

Ernst, Amy A., Steven J. Weiss, Todd G. Nick, Kenneth Iserson, and Michelle H. Biros. "Minimal-Risk Waiver of Informed Consent and Exception from Informed Consent (Final Rule) Studies at Institutional Review Boards Nationwide." *Academic Emergency Medicine* 12, no. 11 (2005): 1134–37.

Espeland, Wendy Nelson. *The Struggle for Water: Politics, Rationality, and Identity in the American Southwest*. Chicago: University of Chicago Press, 1998.

Espeland, Wendy Nelson, and Michael Sauder. "Rankings and Reactivity: How Public Measures Recreate Social Worlds." *American Journal of Sociology* 113, no. 1 (2007): 1–40.

Espeland, Wendy Nelson, and Mitchell L. Stevens. "Commensuration as a Social Process." *Annual Review of Sociology* 24 (1998): 313–43.

Espeland, Wendy Nelson, and Berit Irene Vannebo. "Accountability, Quantification, and Law." *Annual Review of Law and Social Science* 3, no. 1 (2007): 21–43.

Evans, John H. *Playing God? Human Genetic Engineering and the Rationalization of Public Bioethical Debate*. Chicago: University of Chicago Press, 2002.

———. "A Sociological Account of the Growth of Principlism." *Hastings Center Report* 30, no. 5 (2000): 31–38.

Ewick, Patricia, and Susan S. Silbey. *The Common Place of Law: Stories from Everyday Life*. Language and Legal Discourse. Chicago: University of Chicago Press, 1998.

Faden, Ruth R., and Tom L. Beauchamp. *A History and Theory of Informed Consent*. New York: Oxford University Press, 1986.

Fahrenthold, Elsie. "It's a Model Hospital but—Admission to Clinical Center Based on Research Needs." *NIH Record*, January 17, 1961, 1,8.

Farreras, Ingrid, Caroline Hannaway, and Victoria A. Harden, eds. *Mind, Brain, Body, and Behavior: Foundations of Neuroscience and Behavioral Research at the National Institutes of Health*. Washington, DC: IOS Press, 2004.

Feeley, Malcolm M. "Legality, Social Research, and the Challenge of Institutional Review Boards." *Law and Society Review* 41, no. 4 (2007): 757–76.

The Final Report of the Advisory Committee on Human Radiation Experiments. Edited by Experiments Advisory Committee on Human Radiation. New York: Oxford University Press, 1996.

Fine, Gary A. "The Sociology of the Local: Action and Its Publics." *Sociological Theory* 28, no. 4 (2010): 355–76.

Fisher, Jill A. *Medical Research for Hire: The Political Economy of Pharmaceutical Clinical Trials*. Critical Issues in Health and Medicine. New Brunswick, NJ: Rutgers University Press, 2009.

Fletcher, John C. "Location of the Office for the Protection from Research Risks within the National Institutes of Health: Problems of Status and Independent Authority." In *Ethical and Policy Issues in Research Involving Human Participants*, vol. 2. Bethesda, MD: National Bioethics Advisory Commission, 2001.

Forrester, John. "If *p*, Then What? Thinking in Cases." *History of the Human Sciences* 9, no. 3 (1996): 1–25.

———. "The Psychoanalytic Case: Voyeurism, Ethics, and Epistemology in Robert Stoller's *Sexual Excitement*." In *Science without Laws: Model Systems, Cases, Exemplary Narratives*, edited by Angela N. H. Creager, Elizabeth Lunbeck, and M. Norton Wise, 189–211. Durham, NC: Duke University Press, 2007.

Foucault, Michel. *Discipline and Punish: The Birth of the Prison*. Trans. Alan Sheriden. New York: Random House, 1975.

Fox, Daniel M. "The Politics of the NIH Extramural Program, 1937–1950." *Journal of the History of Medicine and Allied Sciences* 42, no. 4 (1987): 447–66.

Frankel, Mark S. "The Development of Policy Guidelines Governing Human Experimentation in the United States: A Case Study of Public Policy-Making for Science and Technology." *Ethics in Science and Medicine* 2, no 1 (1975): 43–59.

Frazer, Heather T., and John O'Sullivan. *We Have Just Begun to Not Fight: An Oral History of Conscientious Objectors in Civilian Public Service during World War II*. Twayne's Oral History Series. New York: Twayne, 1996.

Freidson, Eliot. "The Changing Nature of Professional Control." *Annual Review of Sociology* 10 (1984): 1–20.

Garfinkel, Harold. *Studies in Ethnomethodology*. Englewood Cliffs, NJ: Prentice Hall, 1967.

Geison, Gerald L. "Divided We Stand: Physiologists and Clinicians in the American Context." In *Sickness and Health in America*, edited by Judith W. Leavitt and Ronald L. Numbers, 115–129. Madison: University of Wisconsin Press, 1978.

Gilchrist, Irvin, and Urban Information Interpreters. *Medical Experimentation on Prisoners Must Stop: Documents Generated during the Course of a Struggle*. Urban Information Series Publications 13. College Park, MD.: Urban Information Interpreters, 1974.

Gingerich, Melvin. *Service for Peace: A History of Mennonite Civilian Public Service*. Akron, PA: Mennonite Central Committee, 1949.

Glantz, Leonard H. "The Influence of the Nuremberg Code on US Statutes and Regulations." In *The Nazi Doctors and the Nuremberg Code: Human Rights and Human Experimentation*, edited by George J. Annas and Michael A. Grodin, 183–200. New York: Oxford University Press, 1992.

Goldman, Jerry, and Martin D. Katz. "Inconsistency and Institutional Review Boards." *Journal of the American Medical Association* 248, no. 2 (1982): 197–202.

Goodman, Jordan, Anthony McElligott, and Lara Marks, eds. *Useful Bodies: Humans in the Service of Medical Science in the Twentieth Century*. Baltimore: Johns Hopkins University Press, 2003.

Gostin, Lawrence O., Cori Vanchieri, Andrew MacPherson Pope, Institute of Medicine (U.S.). Committee on Ethical Considerations for Revisions to DHHS Regulations for Protection of Prisoners Involved in Research, and Institute of Medicine (U.S.) Board on Health Sciences Policy. *Ethical Considerations for Research Involving Prisoners*. Washington, DC: National Academies Press, 2007.

Green, Lee A., Julie C. Lowery, Christine P. Kowalski, and Leon Wyszewianski. "Impact of Institutional Review Board Practice Variation on Observational Health Services Research." *Health Services Research* 41, no. 1 (2006): 214–30.

Greenberg, Daniel S. "NIH and Fountain: Part of the Problem Is That an Atmosphere of Suspicion Has Enveloped the Relationship." *Science* 140 (1963): 1076–78.

———. *The Politics of Pure Science*. New ed. Chicago: University of Chicago Press, 1999.

Grieveson, Lee. *Policing Cinema: Movies and Censorship in Early-Twentieth-Century America*. Berkeley: University of California Press, 2004.

Guerrini, Anita. "Human Rights, Animal Rights, and the Conduct of Science." In *Experimenting with Humans and Animals: From Galen to Animal Rights*, by Guerrini, 137–52. Johns Hopkins Introductory Studies in the History of Science. Baltimore: Johns Hopkins University Press, 2003.

Guetzkow, Joshua, Michèle Lamont, and Grégoire Mallard. "What Is Originality in the Humanities and the Social Sciences?" *American Sociological Review* 69, no. 2 (2004): 190–212.

" 'Guinea Pig' Society." *NIH Record*, December 26, 1951.

Gusterson, Hugh. "The Auditors." *Boston Review*, November–December (2005).

Guston, David H. "On Consensus and Voting in Science: From Asilomar to the National Toxicology Program." In *The New Political Sociology of Science: Institutions, Networks, and Power*, edited by Kelly Moore and Scott Frickel, 378–404. Madison: University of Wisconsin Press, 2006.

Gutmann, Amy. "Bureaucracy, Professionalism, and Participation." In *Liberal Equality*, by Gutmann, 201–11. New York: Cambridge University Press, 1980.

Hacking, Ian. *Historical Ontology*. Cambridge, MA: Harvard University Press, 2004.

———. "Making Up People." In *Reconstructing Individualism: Autonomy, Individuality, and the Self in Western Thought*, edited by Thomas C. Heller, Morton Sosna, and David E. Wellbery, 222–36. Stanford, CA: Stanford University Press, 1986.

Haliski, Jenny. "Church Volunteers from 1954–1975 Reunite at Clinical Center." *NIH Record*, November 16, 2007.

Halpern, Sydney. *Lesser Harms: The Morality of Risk in Medical Research*. Chicago: University of Chicago Press, 2004.

Hamilton, Michael. "Some Precision Would Be Helpful." *IRB* 26, no. 5 (2004): 19.

Harkness, Jon. "Research behind Bars: A History of Nontherapeutic Research on American Prisoners." Ph.D. diss., University of Wisconsin, 1996.

———. "The Significance of the Nuremberg Code." *New England Journal of Medicine* 338, no. 14 (1998): 995–96.

Haseltine, Nate. "New Hospital Is Primarily for Research." *Washington Post*, August 9, 1953, B1.

———. "Objectors Aid Clinic Center Health Tests." *Washington Post*, May 26, 1954.

Hedgecoe, Adam. "Research Ethics Review and the Sociological Research Relationship." *Sociology* 42, no. 5 (2008): 873–86.

Heilbron, J. L., and Robert W. Seidel. *Lawrence and His Laboratory: A History of the Lawrence Berkeley Laboratory*. Los Angeles: University of California Press, 1989.

Heimer, Carol A. "Cases and Biographies: An Essay on Routinization and the Nature of Comparison." *Annual Review of Sociology* 27 (2001): 47–76.

Heimer, Carol, and JuLeigh Petty. "Bureaucratic Ethics: IRBs and the Legal Regulation of Human Subjects Research." *Annual Review of Law and Social Science* 6 (2010): 601–26.

Hirshon, Jon Mark, Scott D. Krugman, Michael Witting, Jon Furuno, M. Rhona Limcangco, Andre R. Perisse, and Elizabeth K. Rasch. "Variability in Institutional Review Board Assessment of Minimal-Risk Research." *Academic Emergency Medicine* 9, no. 12 (2008): 1417–20.

Hurlbut, James Benjamin. "Experiments in Democracy: The Science, Politics, and Ethics of Human Embryo Research in the United States, 1978–2007." Ph.D. diss., Harvard University, 2010.

Igo, Sarah E. *The Averaged American: Surveys, Citizens, and the Making of a Mass Public.* Cambridge, MA: Harvard University Press, 2007.

Irvin, Renee A., and John Stansbury. "Citizen Participation in Decision Making: Is It Worth the Effort?" *Public Administration Review* 64 (2004): 55–65.

Jacob, Marie Andrée, and Annelise Riles. "The New Bureaucracies of Virtue: Introduction." *Political and Legal Anthropology Review* 30, no. 2 (2007): 181–91.

Jaeger, Jan. "An Ethnographic Analysis of Institutional Review Board Decision-Making." Ph.D. diss., University of Pennsylvania, 2006.

Jasanoff, Sheila. *Designs on Nature: Science and Democracy in Europe and the United States.* Princeton, NJ: Princeton University Press, 2007.

———. *The Fifth Branch: Science Advisers as Policy Makers.* Cambridge, MA: Harvard University Press, 1990.

———. "Ordering Knowledge, Ordering Society." In *States of Knowledge: The Co-Production of Science and Social Order*, edited by Sheila Jasanoff, 13–45. New York: Routledge, 2004.

———. "Science and the Statistical Victim: Modernizing Knowledge in Breast Implant Litigation." *Social Studies of Science* 32, no. 1 (2002): 37–69.

Jones, David, and Robert Martensen. "Human Radiation Experiments and the Formation of Medical Physics at the University of California, San Francisco and Berkeley, 1937–1962." In Goodman, McElligott, and Marks, *Useful Bodies*, 81–108.

Jones, James. *Bad Blood: The Scandalous Story of the Tuskegee Experiment—When Government Doctors Played God and Science Went Mad.* New York: Maxwell McMillan, 1981.

Junod, Suzanne W. "Highlights in the History of Informed Patient Consent." Unpublished report, FDA History Office, 1998.

Kanigel, Robert. *Apprentice to Genius: The Making of a Scientific Dynasty.* New York: Macmillan, 1986.

Kasel, J. A., R. H. Alford, V. Knight, G. H. Waddell, and M. M. Sigel. "Experimental Infection of Human Volunteers with Equine Influenza Virus." *Nature* 206, no. 4979 (1965): 41.

Katz, Jack. "Toward a Natural History of Ethical Censorship." *Law and Society Review* 41, no. 4 (2007): 797–810.

Katz, Jay. *Experimentation with Human Beings: The Authority of the Investigator, Subject, Professions, and State in the Human Experimentation Process.* New York: Sage, 1972.

———. *The Silent World of Doctor and Patient.* New York: Free Press, 1984.

Katznelson, Ira. "Knowledge about What? Policy Intellectuals and the New Liberalism." In *States, Social Knowledge, and the Origins of Modern Social Policies*, edited by Dietrich Rueschemeyer and Theda Skocpol. New York: Sage; Princeton, NJ: Princeton University Press, 1996.

Keating, Peter, and Alberto Cambrosio. "Who's Minding the Data? Data Monitoring Committees in Clinical Cancer Trials." *Sociology of Health and Illness* 31, no. 3 (2009): 325–42.

Kennedy, Duncan. "The Disenchantment of Logically Formal Legal Rationality, or Max Weber's Sociology in the Genealogy of the Contemporary Mode of Western Legal Thought." *Hastings Law Journal* 55, no. 5 (2004): 1031–76.

Kennedy, Thomas. "James Augustine Shannon." In *Biographical Memoirs*, edited by National Academy of Sciences, 75:356–79. Washington, DC: National Academy Press, 1998.

Kevles, Daniel J. *The Baltimore Case: A Trial of Politics, Science, and Character.* New York: Norton, 1998.

Knight, V. "The Use of Volunteers in Medical Virology." *Progress in Medical Virology* 6 (1964): 1–26.

Koch, Charles H. *Administrative Law and Practice.* 2nd ed., 3 vols. St. Paul, MN: West, 1997.

Kuhn, Thomas S. *The Structure of Scientific Revolutions.* Chicago: University of Chicago Press, 1962.

Kusch, Martin. "Hacking's Historical Epistemology: A Critique of Styles of Reasoning." *Studies in the History and Philosophy of Science* 41, no. 2 (2010): 158–73.

Kutcher, Gerald. *Contested Medicine: Cancer Research and the Military.* Chicago: University of Chicago Press, 2009.

Labott, Susan M., and Timothy P. Johnson. "Psychological and Social Risks of Behavioral Research." *IRB* 26, no. 3 (2004): 11–15.

Ladimer, Irving. "Human Experimentation: Medicolegal Aspects." *New England Journal of Medicine* 257, no. 1 (1957): 18–24.

Ladimer, Irving, and Roger Newman, eds. *Clinical Investigation in Medicine: Legal, Ethical, and Moral Aspects; An Anthology and Bibliography.* Boston: Law-Medicine Research Institute, Boston University, 1963.

Lamont, Michèle. *How Professors Think: Inside the Curious World of Academic Judgment.* Cambridge, MA.: Harvard University Press, 2009.

Lamont, Michèle, and Katri Huutoniemi. "Comparing Customary Rules of Fairness: Evidence of Evaluative Practices in Peer Review Panels." In *Social Knowledge in the Making: Knowledge Making, Use, and Evaluation in the Social Sciences*, edited by Charles Camic, Neil Gross, and Michèle Lamont. Chicago: University of Chicago Press, in press.

Langer, Elinor. "Human Experimentation: New York Verdict Affirms Patient's Rights." *Science* 151, no. 3711 (1966): 663–66.

Lasagna, Louis. "Congress, the FDA, and New Drug Development: Before and After 1962." *Perspectives in Biology and Medicine* 32 (1989): 322–43.

Lasagna, Louis, and John M. von Felsinger. "The Volunteer Subject in Research." *Science* 120, no. 3114 (1954): 359–61.

Latour, Bruno. *Science in Action: How to Follow Scientists and Engineers through Society.* Cambridge, MA: Harvard University Press, 1987.

Law, John. "On STS and Sociology." *Sociological Review* 56, no. 4 (2008): 623–49.

Lederer, Susan E. "Research without Borders: The Origins of the Declaration of Helsinki." In *Twentieth Century Ethics of Human Subjects Research: Historical Perspectives on Values, Practices, and Regulations*, edited by Giovanni Maio and Volker Roelcke, 199–217. Stuttgart, Germany: Franz Steiner Verlag, 2004.

———. *Subjected to Science: Human Experimentation in America before the Second World War.* Baltimore: Johns Hopkins University Press, 1995.

Lederman, Rena. *Anthropology among the Disciplines.* Philadelphia: University of Pennsylvania Press, forthcoming.

Lee, Caroline. "Is There a Place for Private Conversation in Public Dialogue? Comparing

Stakeholder Assessments of Informal Communication in Collaborative Regional Planning." *American Journal of Sociology* 113, no. 1 (2007): 41–96.

Levitan, Sar A., and Robert Taggart. *The Promise of Greatness: The Social Programs of the Last Decade and Their Major Achievements.* Cambridge, MA: Harvard University Press, 1976.

Lipscomb, Carolyn E. "Professional Boundaries and Medical Records Management." *Journal of the Medical Library Association* 91, no. 4 (2003): 393–96.

Lipsky, Michael. *Street-Level Bureaucracy: Dilemmas of the Individual in Public Services.* 1980. 30th anniversary expanded ed. New York: Sage, 2010.

Loh, E. D., and R. E. Meyer. "Medical Schools' Attitudes and Perceptions regarding the Use of Central Institutional Review Boards." *Academic Medicine* 79, no. 7 (2004): 644–51.

Lyons, Michele. *70 Acres of Science: The National Institute of Health Moves to Bethesda.* www.history.nih.gov/01Docs/historical/documents/70AcresofSciencejuly14.pdf, NIH, 2006. Accessed February 2010.

MacKenzie, Donald A., Fabian Muniesa, and Lucia Siu. *Do Economists Make Markets? On the Performativity of Economics.* Princeton, NJ: Princeton University Press, 2007.

Mackenzie, G. Calvin, and Robert Weisbrot. "The Federal Colossus." In *The Liberal Hour: Washington and the Politics of Change in the 1960s.* New York: Penguin Press, 2008.

Mallard, Grégoire, Michèle Lamont, and Joshua Guetzkow. "Fairness as Appropriateness: Negotiating Epistemological Differences in Peer Review." *Science, Technology, and Human Values* 34, no. 5 (2009): 573–606.

Mandel, Richard. "Beacon of Hope: The Clinical Center through Forty Years of Growth and Change." National Institutes of Health, http://history.nih.gov/exhibits/beacon/.

Marks, Harry M. "The 1954 Salk Poliomyelitis Vaccine Field Trial." In *100 Landmark Clinical Trials,* edited by Marks, Goodman, and Robinson. Wiley, Forthcoming.

———. *The Progress of Experiment: Science and Therapeutic Reform in the United States, 1900–1990.* Cambridge: Cambridge University Press, 1997.

———. "Trust and Mistrust in the Marketplace: Statistics and Clinical Research, 1945–1960." *History of Science* 38 (2000): 343–55.

Marks, John. *The Search for the Manchurian Candidate: The CIA and Mind Control.* New York: Norton, 1991.

Martensen, Robert. "The History of Bioethics: An Essay Review." *Journal of the History of Medicine and Allied Sciences* 56, no. 2 (2001): 168–75.

Martin, Emily. *Bipolar Expeditions: Mania and Depression in American Culture.* Princeton, NJ: Princeton University Press, 2007.

McCarthy, Charles. "The Origins and Policies That Govern Institutional Review Boards." In *The Oxford Textbook on Clinical Research Ethics,* edited by Ezekiel Emanuel, Christine Grady, Robert A. Crouch, Reidar K. Lie, Franklin G. Miller, and David Wedler. New York: Oxford University Press, 2008.

———. "Reflections on the Organizational Locus of the Office for the Protection from Research Risks." In *Ethical and Policy Issues in Research Involving Human Participants,* vol. 2. Bethesda, MD: National Bioethics Advisory Commission, 2001.

McWilliams, Rita, Julie Hoover-Fong, Ada Hamosh, Suzanne Beck, Terri Beaty, and Garry Cutting. "Problematic Variation in Local Institutional Review of a Multicenter Genetic Epidemiology Study." *Journal of the American Medical Association* 290, no. 3 (2003): 360–66.

Menikoff, Jerry. "The Paradoxical Problem with Multiple-IRB Review." *New England Journal of Medicine* 363 (2010): 1591–93.

Moreno, Jonathan D. *Deciding Together: Bioethics and Moral Consensus.* Oxford: Oxford University Press, 1995.

———. "Reassessing the Influence of the Nuremberg Code on American Medical Ethics." *Journal of Contemporary Health Law and Policy* 13, no. 2 (1997): 347–60.

———. *Undue Risk: Secret State Experiments on Humans.* New York: Routledge, 2001.

Mukerji, Chandra. *A Fragile Power: Scientists and the State.* Princeton, NJ: Princeton University Press, 1989.

Mullan, Fitzhugh. *Plagues and Politics: The Story of the United States Public Health Service.* New York: Basic Books, 1989.

Nathan, David G. "Careers in Translational Clinical Research: Historical Perspectives, Future Challenges." *Journal of the American Medical Association* 287, no. 18 (2002): 2424–27.

National Bioethics Advisory Commission. "Ethical and Policy Issues in Research Involving Human Participants, Vol. I." National Bioethics Advisory Commission, Washington, DC, 2001.

"NIH Radiation Safety Experts Test Switchboard." *NIH Record,* May 25, 1953.

"Normal Volunteers Take Part in Research." *NIH Record,* June 21, 1954.

Novak, Steven J. "LSD before Leary: Sidney Cohen's Critique of 1950s Psychedelic Drug Research." *Isis* 88, no. 1 (1997): 87–110.

Offit, Paul A. *The Cutter Incident: How America's First Polio Vaccine Led to the Growing Vaccine Crisis.* New Haven, CT: Yale University Press, 2005.

Pager, Devah. *Marked: Race, Crime, and Finding Work in an Era of Mass Incarceration.* Chicago: University of Chicago Press, 2007.

Park, Buhm Soon. "The Development of the Intramural Research Program at the National Institutes of Health after World War II." *Perspectives in Biology and Medicine* 46, no. 3 (2003): 383–402.

Petryna, Adriana. *When Experiments Travel: Clinical Trials and the Global Search for Human Subjects.* Princeton, NJ: Princeton University Press, 2009.

Polletta, Francesca. *Freedom Is an Endless Meeting: Democracy in American Social Movements.* Chicago: University of Chicago Press, 2002.

———. *It Was like a Fever: Storytelling in Protest and Politics.* Chicago: University of Chicago Press, 2006.

Polletta, Francesca, and John Lee. "Is Telling Stories Good for Democracy? Rhetoric in Public Deliberation after 9/11." *American Sociological Review* 71, no. 5 (2006): 699–721.

Pollin, W., and S. Perlin. "Psychiatric Evaluation of 'Normal Control' Volunteers." *American Journal of Psychiatry* 115 (1958): 129–33.

Porter, Theodore. *Trust in Numbers: The Pursuit of Objectivity in Science and Public Life.* Princeton, NJ: Princeton University Press, 1995.

Powell, Walter W., and Paul DiMaggio. *The New Institutionalism in Organizational Analysis.* Chicago: University of Chicago Press, 1991.

"Practice Runs at NIH Show Progress." "Civil Defense" issue of *NIH Record,* May 14, 1952.

Prescott, Heather Munro. "Using the Student Body: College and University Students as Research Subjects in the United States during the Twentieth Century." *Journal of the History of Medicine and Allied Sciences* 57, no. 1 (2002): 3–38.

Rabeharisoa, Vololona, and Michel Callon. "Patients and Scientists in French Muscular Dystrophy Research." In *States of Knowledge: The Co-Production of Science and Social Order,* edited by Sheila Jasanoff, 142–60. London: Routledge, 2004.

Reardon, Jenny. "Creating Participatory Subjects: Science, Race, and Democracy in a Genomic Age." In *The New Political Sociology of Science,* edited by Scott Frickel and Kelly Moore, 351–77. Madison: University of Wisconsin Press, 2006.

————. *Race to the Finish: Identity and Governance in an Age of Genomics*. Princeton, NJ: Princeton University Press, 2005.

Rector, Thomas S. "How Should We Communicate the Likelihood of Risks to Inform Decisions about Consent?" *IRB* 30, no. 4 (2008): 15–18.

Reed, Adam. "Documents Unfolding." In *Documents: Artifacts of Modern Knowledge*, edited by Annelise Riles, 158–79. Ann Arbor: University of Michigan Press, 2006.

Reverby, Susan. *Examining Tuskegee: The Infamous Syphilis Study and Its Legacy*. John Hope Franklin Series in African American History and Culture. Chapel Hill: University of North Carolina Press, 2009.

————. "'Normal Exposure' and Inoculation Syphilis: A PHS 'Tuskegee' Doctor in Guatemala, 1946–48." *Journal of Policy History* 23, no. 1 (2010): 6–28.

Risse, G. B., and J. H. Warner. "Reconstructing Clinical Activities: Patient Records in Medical History." *Social History of Medicine* 5, no. 2 (1992): 183–205.

Roelcke, Volker, and Giovanni Maio, eds. *Twentieth Century Ethics of Human Subjects Research: Historical Perspectives on Values, Practices, and Regulations*. Stuttgart: Franz Steiner, 2004.

Rose, Nikolas. *Inventing Ourselves: Psychology, Power, and Personhood*. New York: Cambridge University Press, 1998.

Rosenberg, Charles. *The Care of Strangers: The Rise of America's Hospital System*. New York: Basic Books, 1987.

Rossiter, Margaret W. *Women Scientists in America: Before Affirmative Action, 1940–1972*. Baltimore: Johns Hopkins University Press, 1995.

Rothman, David. *Strangers at the Bedside: A History of How Law and Bioethics Transformed Medical Decisionmaking*. New York: Basic Books, 1991.

Rourke, Edward J. "Experimentation in Children." *Journal of the American Medical Association* 211, no. 2 (1970): 301.

Savage, Charles. "Lysergic Acid Diethylamide (LSD-25): A Clinical-Psychological Study." *American Journal of Psychiatry* 108 (1952): 896–900.

Schechter, Alan N. "The Crisis in Clinical Research: Endangering the Half Century National Institutes of Health Consensus." *Journal of the American Medical Association* 280, no. 16 (1998): 1440–42.

Schiebinger, Londa. "Human Experimentation in the Eighteenth Century: Natural Boundaries and Valid Testing." In *The Moral Authority of Nature*, edited by Lorraine Daston and Fernando Vidal, 384–408. Chicago: University of Chicago Press, 2004.

Schrag, Zachary M. *Ethical Imperialism: Institutional Review Boards and the Social Sciences, 1965–2009*. Baltimore: Johns Hopkins University Press, 2010.

————. "How Talking Became Human Subjects Research: The Federal Regulation of the Social Sciences, 1965–1991." *Journal of Policy History* 21, no. 1 (2009): 3–37.

Scientists' Committee on Loyalty and Security. "Loyalty and US Public Health Service Grants." *Bulletin of the Atomic Sciences* 11, no. 5 (1955): 196–97.

Scott, James C. *Seeing like a State: How Certain Schemes to Improve the Human Condition Have Failed*. Yale Agrarian Studies. New Haven, CT: Yale University Press, 1998.

Shannon, James A. "Clinical Testing of Antimalarial Drugs." In *Advances in Military Medicine, Made by American Investigators*, edited by United States Office of Scientific Research and Development, Committee on Medical Research, and Edwin Cowles Andrus, 698–716. 2 vols. Boston: Little, Brown, 1948.

————. "The National Institutes of Health: Programmes and Problems." *Proceedings of the Royal Society of London, Series B, Biological Sciences* 155 (1961): 171–82.

———. "The National Institutes of Health: Some Critical Years, 1955–1957." *Science* 237, no. 4817 (1987): 865–68.

Shapin, Steven. *The Scientific Life: A Moral History of a Late Modern Vocation.* Chicago: University of Chicago Press, 2008.

———. *A Social History of Truth: Civility and Science in Seventeenth-Century England.* Science and Its Conceptual Foundation. Chicago: University of Chicago Press, 1994.

———. "Trusting George Cheyne: Scientific Expertise, Common Sense, and Moral Authority in Early Eighteenth-Century Dietetic Medicine." *Bulletin of the History of Medicine* 77, no. 2 (2003): 263–97.

Shapin, Steven, and Christopher Lawrence. "Introduction: The Body of Knowledge." In *Science Incarnate*, edited by Steven Shapin, 1–19. Chicago: University of Chicago Press, 1998.

Shapin, Steven, and Simon Schaffer. *Leviathan and the Air-Pump: Hobbes, Boyle, and the Experimental Life.* Princeton, NJ: Princeton University Press, 1985.

Shimkin, Michael. "Scientific Investigations on Man: A Medical Research Worker's Viewpoint." In *Biomedical Ethics and the Law*, edited by James Humber and Robert Almeder, 229–38. New York: Springer, 1979.

Shore, Chris, and Susan Wright. "Coercive Accountability." In *Audit Cultures: Anthropological Studies in Accountability, Ethics, and the Academy*, edited by Marilyn Strathern, 57–89. London: Routledge, 2000.

Silverman, Henry, Sara Candros Hull, and Jeremy Sugarman. "Variability among Institutional Review Boards' Decisions within the Context of a Multicenter Trial." *Critical Care Medicine* 29, no. 2 (2001): 235–41.

Skrentny, John D. *The Minority Rights Revolution.* Cambridge, MA: Harvard University Press, 2002.

Smith, Dorothy E. "Incorporating Texts into Ethnographic Practice." In *Institutional Ethnography as Practice*, edited by Dorothy E. Smith, 65–88. New York: Rowman and Littlefield, 2006.

Smith, Frank. "1000th Prisoner Volunteer Admitted to Clinical Center." *NIH Record*, August 25, 1964.

Spearin, Carole. "CC Medical Record Dept. Processes Information Vital to Clinical Research." *NIH Record*, November 7, 1961, 2.

Stair, Thomas O., Caitlin R. Reed, Michael S. Radeos, Greg Koski, and Carlos A. Camargo. "Variation in Institutional Review Board Responses to a Standard Protocol for a Multicenter Trial." *Academic Emergency Medicine* 8, no. 6 (2001): 636–41.

Stark, Laura. "The Science of Ethics: Deception, the Resilient Self, and the APA Code of Ethics, 1966–1973." *Journal of the History of the Behavioral Sciences* 46, no. 4 (2010): 337–70.

———. "Victims in Our Own Minds? IRBs in Myth and Practice." *Law and Society Review* 41, no. 4 (2007): 777–86.

Stark, Laura, and Erin Kelly. "Review of *Professional Guinea Pig.*" *Bulletin of the History of Medicine*, forthcoming.

Stark, Laura, and Eliana Theodorou. "Hospital Architecture and Postwar Theories of Disease: The Case of the NIH Clinical Center." Unpublished paper, 2010.

Starr, Paul. *The Social Transformation of American Medicine.* New York: Basic Books, 1982.

Stevens, Mitchell L. *Creating a Class: College Admissions and the Education of Elites.* Cambridge, MA: Harvard University Press, 2007.

Stevens, Rosemary. *In Sickness and in Wealth: American Hospitals in the Twentieth Century.* New York: Basic Books, 1989.

Strathern, Marilyn. "New Accountabilities: Anthropological Studies in Audit, Ethics, and the Academy." In *Audit Cultures: Anthropological Studies in Accountability, Ethics, and the Academy*, edited by Marilyn Strathern, 1–18. London: Routledge, 2000.

Strickland, Stephen P. *Politics, Science, and Dread Disease: A Short History of United States Medical Research Policy*. Cambridge, MA: Harvard University Press, 1972.

Stryker, Robin. "Rules, Resources, and Legitimacy Processes: Some Implications for Social Conflict, Order, and Change." *American Journal of Sociology* 99, no. 4 (1994): 847–910.

"Studies on Radiation Biology." *NIH Record*, August 29, 1949, 2.

Suchman, Mark C. "The Contract as Social Artifact." *Law and Society* 37, no. 1 (2003): 91–142.

Sunstein, Cass R. *Worst-Case Scenarios*. Cambridge, MA: Harvard University Press, 2007.

Taylor, Holly A., Peter Currie, and Nancy E. Kass. "A Study to Evaluate the Effect of Investigator Attendance on the Efficiency of IRB Review." *IRB* 30, no. 1 (2008): 1–5.

Thorpe, Charles, and Steven Shapin. "Who Was J. Robert Oppenheimer? Charisma and Complex Organization." *Social Studies of Science* 30, no. 4 (2000): 545–90.

Timmermans, Stefan. *Postmortem: How Medical Examiners Explain Suspicious Deaths*. Chicago: University of Chicago Press, 2006.

Timmermans, Stefan, and Marc Berg. *The Gold Standard: The Challenge of Evidence-Based Medicine and Standardization in Health Care*. Philadelphia: Temple University Press, 2003.

Titunik, Regina F. "Democracy, Domination, and Legitimacy in Max Weber's Political Thought." In *Max Weber's Economy and Society*, edited by Charles Camic, Philip S. Gorski, and David M. Trubek, 143–63. Stanford, CA: Stanford University Press, 2005.

Tobbell, Dominique A. "Allied against Reform: Pharmaceutical Industry–Academic Physician Relations in the United States, 1945–1970." *Bulletin of the History of Medicine* 82, no. 4 (2008): 878–912.

Topping, Norman. *Recollections*. Los Angeles: University of Southern California, 1990.

———. "The United States Public Health Service's Clinical Center for Medical Research." *Journal of the American Medical Association* 150, no. 6 (1952): 541–45.

Toulmin, S. "How Medicine Saved the Life of Ethics." *Perspectives in Biology and Medicine* 25, no. 4 (1982): 736–50.

———. "The Layout of Arguments." In *The Uses of Argument*, 87–134. Cambridge: Cambridge University Press, 2003.

Tracy, Sarah. "Fasting for Research and Relief: Ancel Keys and the Minnesota Starvation Experiment, 1945–1946." Paper presented at Annual Meeting of the American Association for the History of Medicine, Rochester, MN, May 2, 2010.

Tsay, Angela, Michèle Lamont, Andrew Abbott, and Joshua Guetzkow. "From Character to Intellect: Changing Conceptions of Merit in the Social Sciences and Humanities, 1951–1971." *Poetics* 31 (2003): 23–49.

Tucker, Todd. *The Great Starvation Experiment: Ancel Keys and the Men Who Starved for Science*. 1st University of Minnesota Press ed. Minneapolis: University of Minnesota Press, 2007.

Turner, Stephen. "What Is the Problem with Experts?" *Social Studies of Science* 31, no. 1 (2001): 123–49.

Vaughan, Diane. *The Challenger Launch Decision: Risky Technology, Culture, and Deviance at NASA*. Chicago: University of Chicago Press, 1996.

Veatch, Robert M. *The Patient as Partner: A Theory of Human Experimentation Ethics*. Bloomington: Indiana University Press, 1987.

Waddell, Craig. "Reasonableness versus Rationality in the Construction and Justification of Science Policy Decisions: The Case of the Cambridge Experimentation Review Board." *Science, Technology, and Human Values* 14, no. 1 (1989): 7–25.

Wagner, T. H., C. Murray, J. Goldberg, J. M. Adler, and J. Abrams. "Costs and Benefits of the National Cancer Institute Central Institutional Review Board." *Journal of Clinical Oncology* 28 (2010): 662–66.

Wang, Jessica. *American Science in an Age of Anxiety: Scientists, Anticommunism, and the Cold War.* Chapel Hill: University of North Carolina Press, 1999.

Washington, Harriet A. *Medical Apartheid: The Dark History of Medical Experimentation on Black Americans from Colonial Times to the Present.* 1st ed. New York: Doubleday, 2006.

Weber, Max. *Economy and Society.* Edited by Guenther Roth and Claus Wittich. Vol. 2. Berkeley: University of California Press, 1978.

Weindling, Paul. "The Origins of Informed Consent: The International Scientific Commission on Medical War Crimes, and the Nuremberg Code." *Bulletin of the History of Medicine* 75, no. 1 (2001): 37–71.

Welsome, Eileen. *The Plutonium Files: America's Secret Medical Experiments in the Cold War.* New York: Dial Press, 1999.

Wilde, Melissa J. *Vatican II: A Sociological Analysis of Religious Change.* Princeton, NJ: Princeton University Press, 2007.

Williams, Gareth, and Jennie Popay. "Lay Knowledge and the Privilege of Experience." In *Challenging Medicine,* edited by Jonathan Gabe, David Kelleher, and Gareth Williams, 118–40. London: Routledge, 1994.

Wolfle, Dael. "Achievement and Management." *Science* 158 (1967): 721.

Wood, Anne, Christine Grady, and Ezekiel Emanuel. "Regional Ethics Organizations for Protection of Human Research Participants." *Nature Medicine* 10 (2004): 1283–88.

Wood, Christine V. "The Sociologies of Knowledge, Science, and Intellectuals: Distinctive Traditions and Overlapping Perspectives." *Sociology Compass* 4, no. 10 (2010): 909–23.

Wuthnow, Robert. "Promoting Social Trust." In *Saving America?* by Wuthnow, 235–55. Princeton, NJ: Princeton University Press, 2006.

———. "Trust as an Aspect of Social Structure." In *Self, Social Structure, and Beliefs: Explorations in Sociology,* edited by Jeffrey C. Alexander, Gary T. Marx, and Christine L. Williams, 145–67. Berkeley: University of California Press, 2004.

Wyatt, R. G., R. Dolin, N. R. Blacklow, H. L. DuPont, R. F. Buscho, T. S. Thornhil, A. Z. Kapikian, and R. M. Chanock. "Comparison of Three Agents of Acute Infectious Nonbacterial Gastroenteritis by Cross-Challenge in Volunteers." *Journal of Infectious Diseases* 129, no. 6 (1974): 709–14.

Wyatt, Richard. "Commentary on Stark: 'Ethics at "The Ideal Hospital of the Future": How the NIH Clinical Center Changed American Research Ethics.'" Paper presented at the Stetten Symposium on History in the NIH, Bethesda, MD, June 16, 2009.

Wynne, Brian. "May the Sheep Safely Graze? A Reflexive View of the Expert-Lay Knowledge Divide." In *Risk, Environment, and Modernity: Towards a New Ecology,* edited by Scott Lash, Bronislaw Szerszynski, and Brian Wynne, 44–83. New York: Sage, 1996.

Morality and Society Series

EDITED BY ALAN WOLFE

For the Sake of the Children: The Social Organization of Responsibility in the Hospital and the Home
CAROL A. HEIMER AND LISA R. STAFFEN

Money, Morals, and Manners: The Culture of the French and the American Upper-Middle Class
MICHÈLE LAMONT

Streets of Glory: Church and Community in a Black Urban Neighborhood
OMAR MAURICE MCROBERTS

...tion Works

G... *...ion in Black America*

T... *...nd the United States*

...Life

...Women

...America

...d Dichotomy
...R

...sbands

...erica